I·N·N·E·R
CLEANSING

How to Free Yourself From
Joint-Muscle-Artery-Circulation Sludge

REVISED AND EXPANDED

CARLSON WADE

PREN

Paramus,

D1166736

Library of Congress Cataloging-in-Publication Data

Wade, Carlson
 Inner cleansing : how to free yourself from joint-muscle-artery–circulation sludge /
Carlson Wade. — Rev. and expanded.
  p. cm.
 Includes bibliographical references and index.
 ISBN 0-13-474586-8. — ISBN 0-13-474594-9 (pbk.)
 1. Nutrition. 2. Auto-intoxication. 3. Rejuvenation. 4. Enzymes—Therapeutic
use. I. Title.
 RA784.W255 1992
 615.8′54—dc20
                            92-7937
                              CIP

Printed in the United States of America

10 9 8 7

This book is a reference work based on research by the author. The opinions expressed
herein are not necessarily those of or endorsed by the publisher. The directions stated in
this book are in no way to be considered as a substitute for consultation with a duly
licensed doctor.

ISBN 0-13-474586-8 ISBN 0-13-474594-9 (pbk)

ATTENTION: CORPORATIONS AND SCHOOLS

Prentice Hall books are available at quantity discounts with bulk purchase for
educational, business, or sales promotional use. For information, please write to:
Prentice Hall Career & Personal Development Special Sales, 240 Frisch Court,
Paramus, New Jersey 07652. Please supply: title of book, ISBN number, quantity,
how the book will be used, date needed.

 PRENTICE HALL
Career & Personal Development
Paramus, NJ 07652
A Simon & Schuster Company

On the World Wide Web at http://www.phdirect.com

Prentice-Hall International (UK) Limited, *London*
Prentice-Hall of Australia Pty. Limited, *Sydney*
Prentice-Hall Canada Inc., *Toronto*
Prentice-Hall Hispanoamericana, S.A., *Mexico*
Prentice-Hall of India Private Limited, *New Delhi*
Prentice-Hall of Japan, Inc., *Tokyo*
Simon & Schuster Asia Pte. Ltd., *Singapore*
Editora Prentice-Hall do Brasil, Ltda., *Rio de Janeiro*

Dedication

To Your Sparkling Clean and
Youthful New Body and Mind

About the Author

Carlson Wade, one of the nation's foremost medical-nutrition reporters, has written 26 books in the field of natural healing. He writes for many magazines, newspapers, and makes dozens of radio, television, and personal appearances every year. He is a columnist for the Nutrition and Dietary Consultant Journal, and hundreds of Mr. Wade's features and medical news columns have been published in countries world-wide, including France, Spain, Germany, and Japan. He is an accredited member of the American Medical Writers Association and the National Association of Science Writers.

OTHER BOOKS BY THE AUTHOR

Help Yourself With New Enzyme Catalyst Health Secrets

Eat Away Illness: How To Age-Proof Your Body With Anti-Oxidant Foods

Nutritional Healers: How To Eat Your Way To Better Health

How To Beat Arthritis With Immune Power Boosters

Immune Power Boosters: Your Key To Feeling Younger, Living Longer

The Home Encyclopedia Of Symptoms, Ailments And Their Natural Remedies

Foreword

Suddenly, there is a bright new world of youthful health. It is yours, ready for the taking.

This was my immediate reaction when I read Carlson Wade's updated, revised, and expanded book, *Inner Cleansing: How to Free Yourself From Joint-Muscle-Artery-Circulation Sludge.* He offers you a step-by-step set of programs to self-rejuvenation from head to toe. In this age of pollution—from the environment to the foods you eat—this surely is a dynamic key to speedy detoxification, the body makeover that will rebuild your youth . . . from the inside to the outside.

This leading medical reporter has uncovered the basic causes of hundreds of common and uncommon problems, including: premature aging, allergies, digestive disorders, cardiovascular complaints, overweight, sluggish circulation, high cholesterol, and hurtful aches. All are thoroughly described, followed by amazingly simple but speedily effective home remedies that will detoxify your body and mind, often in a matter of moments. This is a livesaving book!

Carlson Wade calls the problem "internal sludge." He is correct. It is this invisible internal toxic accumulation of wastes that threaten to cause erosion of your body and mind. Toxemia is a major cause of aging. So I am glad that Carlson Wade has "unmasked" this sneak thief of health and life. I highly recommend the easy to follow programs that help you wash pollution right out of your system so you can become sparkling clean and youthfully healthy . . . at any age.

The great joy is that so many of these easy-to-follow home programs give rejuvenation within minutes! I have seen this myself. Carlson Wade presents simple programs that can solve a lifetime of problems immediately. And all are natural. *No* drugs. *No* medicines. *No* hospitalization. You'll never have a sick day. This is truly a miracle in rejuvenation and healing. And it works!

Inner Cleansing is the most helpful book on total healing I have yet to see. I am delighted that it has been updated with the most current rejuvenation discoveries to be of valuable help to everyone. Use it. Discover how it can make you look and feel young again . . . forever.

H W. Holderby, M.D.

What This Book Will Do For You

This updated, revised, and expanded edition was written to alert you to an "invisible" threat to your youthful health. New research has identified it as *toxemia* or "body pollution."

This internal pollution is so deceptive, its gnawing presence is hardly noticed until you start to experience one "hopeless" problem after another. Examples of toxemia range from arthritis to sagging skin, from high blood pressure to clogged arteries, from chronic indigestion to unsightly overweight. What is going wrong? You have allowed toxic wastes to take root inside your body: the aging process is stealthily approaching to overtake your body and mind. Something must be done, and quickly.

This book has been expanded to reveal the latest bio-nutritional discoveries of "body pollution." It zeroes in on the problem of toxemia—why it happens and how you can boost your immune system to cleanse away age-causing pollutants. This newly expanded edition shows how you can reverse the tide of aging and rid yourself of toxic threats to your youthfulness.

All together, in one comprehensive volume, at your fingertips, for immediate use and help, are easy-to-follow programs. They can help add years of vitality to your life. They can restore youth to your body and mind. They can save your life!

This book shows how you can cleanse yourself of many, many common and uncommon toxic ailments—in the privacy of your home. There are *no* drugs, *no* expensive hospitalization costs, *no* cumbersome equipment. Many of the sludge-cleansing detoxification programs are totally free. Some require everyday ingredients that are probably in your pantry right now. All of these inner cleansing programs work amazingly fast. They search out, dissolve, and then wash away internal sediment that might otherwise deteriorate and age your vital systems.

Stiffened by arthritis? Troubled with cholesterol-clogged arteries? Wrinkled skin? Nagging stomach disorders? Stubborn overweight? Choking allergies? Cardiovascular hurts? Blood sludge? Feel aged because of "muscular stiffness"? Then get ready to claim victory over these toxic threats to your health. Follow the easy programs (they're fun, too!) and free your body from pollutants. Detoxification will make you feel young and clean, inside and outside. This book will help you whether these conditions are new or have plagued you for years.

Concerned about the side effects of drugs? About the uncertainties of surgery? The spiralling costs of medical care? Then this expanded edition holds special value. The programs described are *all natural*, and can be done right at home. Often, they cost only pennies (yes, pennies!). Many are free! Most important, they give you detoxification and healing in only a short time. In many situations, you'll see and feel the rejuvenation within minutes! And that is only the start of these benefits.

When these discoveries begin to heal you, say goodbye to hundreds of formerly "hopeless" problems. Discover the joys of looking and feeling young and healthy forever. Reason? This updated, revised edition unmasks the newly discovered basic cause of aging and illness: *internal pollution*. It shows you how to uproot, loosen, and wash away toxic sludge and feel the joys of vigorous, youthful health. You can look younger and live longer with easy detoxification.

How soon will you enjoy this "fountain of youth"? Almost immediately, when you turn the page . . .

Carlson Wade

CONTENTS

Chapter 1

FREE YOURSELF FROM "ARTHRITIS PAIN" WITH BIOLOGICAL WASHING

Free yourself from painful, oft-crippling arthritis by correcting the cause. With the use of simple and effective home programs you can uproot, dislodge, and eliminate internal congestion, often to blame for arthritis pain. These programs of "biological washing" free your neuro-muscular-skeletal system from toxic wastes—those irritating, grating, inflammation-causing leftover accumulations that are largely responsible for arthritis distress. Once these cell-clogging wastes have been washed out of your system, your neuro-muscular-skeletal network functions smoothly. Gone is the blockage that is responsible for the stiffness and pain that grows worse as toxic wastes accumulate.

Arthritis: Why It Happens, Why It Hurts

The word *arthritis* means joint inflammation (*arthr* = joint; *itis* = inflammation). There are more than 100 different types of arthritis. The two major types are:

Osteoarthritis

A degenerative joint disease, osteoarthritis often begins because of joint injury, toxic infestation, or overuse. Weightbearing joints such as the knee, hip, and spine are attacked by wastes and begin to hurt. Corrosive and deteriorating toxic sludge causes osteoarthritic damage: the cartilage surface covering the bone ends becomes rough and eventually wears away. In some cases, an abnormal bone growth called a "spur" can develop. Pain and swelling result from joint inflammation. Continued use of the toxin-infected joint produces more pain.

Rheumatoid Arthritis

This is a chronic condition that affects many body parts, including the joint. Basically, the joint fluid becomes contaminated with wastes that attack the joint surface and cause damage. Inflammation occurs. The joints most commonly involved are those in the hands, wrists, feet, and ankles, but large joints such as hips, knees, and elbows can also be attacked by toxic sludge. Swelling, pain, and stiffness are present, even when the joint is not used. Many joints of the body may be involved at the same time.

Arthritis does have a cause—the toxic sludge that has attacked your basic immune system. Oxygen molecules called "free radicals" are constantly attacking your body. These toxic molecules—breathed in from the atmosphere or generated by your body itself—set off a wave of tissue-bone destruction that, in large part, triggers arthritis and other degenerative conditions. Correct this cause with inner cleansing and you help free yourself from arthritis!

TOXIC WASTE OVERLOAD—ARTHRITIS CAUSE

What Are Toxic Wastes?

Toxic wastes are leftover fragments of incompleted digestive processes; they are remnants from unhealthy foods, refined products, and harsh chemical additives. It is a fact that these harmful "free radical" molecules are everywhere: in the air you breathe, the water you drink, the food you eat, the clothes you wear. The environment, once familiar and respected, is becoming an enemy as toxic chemicals invade the atmosphere, lakes, oceans, soil, and your body!

Toxic wastes become stored throughout your body, in your glands, in your cells. These free radicals circulate throughout your bloodstream. They cling together, creating barriers that prevent free and flexible movement of your limbs and muscles. If these wastes take hold, they trigger arthritis-like distress.

Internally, you become "clogged" or "choked" with these toxic wastes. DANGER: If not washed out, toxic wastes continue accumulating until they damage your joint structure, hurtful inflammation strikes, and you fall victim to what is considered creeping arthritis. Your body has been invaded, and destruction is felt as arthritis in one form or another. Must this happen? Can you prevent or reverse this threat? Yes, with simple, swift *internal washing*—a do-it-yourself detoxification program that uses everyday foods and methods that actually scrub away this pain-causing sludge.

"WASH AWAY ARTHRITIS" WITH THIS TWO-DAY RAW FOOD DETOXIFICATION PLAN

Fresh raw fruits and vegetables (and their fresh juices) are highly concentrated sources of catalytic (scrubbing) enzymes. These enzymes are protein-like substances that initiate a cell-washing action that breaks down, dissolves, and ultimately eliminates the toxic free-radical wastes that irritate your joint-muscle system and are to blame for arthritis distress. To fight back, fresh fruits and vegetables (almost overnight) begin a biological washing of your debris-laden organs and systems. Once free of these blockages, your joints and muscles start to move without hurtful obstruction. Increased flexibility and freedom from arthritis is your reward for internal cleansing.

Simple Two-Day Raw Food Detoxification Plan

Set aside two days per week for this inner cleansing or detoxification plan. During these days, consume nothing but raw foods. *Example:* Eat fresh fruits in any desired combination such as fresh fruits and juices for breakfast and a raw vegetable platter with a vegetable juice for lunch. Dinner could be another raw vegetable meal and any desired vegetable juice. For snacks choose either fresh fruits or raw vegetable chunks.

Detoxification Benefit

Catalytic enzymes in the raw foods are able to devote full activity to dissolving the sludge that has accumulated throughout your body. Without interference from cooked foods, the enzymes work swiftly, breaking down these plaque-like molecules and preparing them for elimination. This simple two-day plan helps undo the wrongdoings of the rest of the week through a welcome detoxification of hurtful free radicals. *Remedy:* Eliminate your consumption of refined and processed foods and cut down on intake of free-radical wastes. You will help establish a more youthful metabolism and inner cleansing rhythm that will free you from the arthritis-causing cellular wastes and toxemia.

CASE HISTORY—"Body Spring Cleaning" Heals Lifetime Arthritis Pain

Pain-wracked fingers that could hardly hold a spoon, a stiff back that made getting up from a chair or bed a painful ordeal, and knees that refused to bend at will so depressed Edna J. that she felt there was no alternative but a hospital or sanatorium. A nutrition-minded nurse looked over her charts and tests and recognized the symptoms of sludge-laden joints and free radical-infected muscles. She told Edna J. to follow a "body spring cleaning" program for only two or even three days each week. It called for eating only raw foods and drinking raw juices in any quantity or combination throughout the day. She was to avoid anything processed or cooked. Edna J. was so desperate, she would try anything. By the end of the second day, she felt her fingers becoming more flexible. She could even bend her knees. Encouraged, she continued on the program for five consecutive days. At the end of the fifth day, she could bend at the waist, do long-neglected housework, even go bowling . . . and win! This simple detoxification program ended her lifetime "hopeless" arthritis pain. To maintain "body spring cleaning" all year long, Edna J. goes on a tasty raw food plan for two days every week. She is rewarded with the flexibility of a youngster. She feels she has been "saved" from the unpleasant future of confinement in a sanatorium . . . thanks to this cellular cleansing detoxification program.

OVERCOME "HOPELESS" ARTHRITIS WITH A NIGHTSHADE-FREE PROGRAM

A group of foods that appear innocent can harbor harmful substances that cause toxic overload. They belong to the nightshade family. These crop plants ordinarily offer good nutriton, but for certain people they become antagonistic. These nightshade foods contain substances which prevent enzymes in your muscles from working to detoxify, cleanse, and wash out waste materials.

Problem

The nightshade foods release toxins which set off the release of *solanine.* Solanine is a crystalline alkaloid which festers in the joints and muscles, causing a sludge buildup, to eventually create enervation (lowered resistance and a weakening of the immune system) and the onset of arthritic distress. Certain people are especially sensitive to even small amounts of solanine. Furthermore, if your metabolism is sluggish, the solanine accumulates and forms a sludge-like toxic barrier in your joint-muscle cells. Blockage is felt in the form of stiff and unyielding joints. Pain, unhappily, is the symptom most often experienced. This can be traced back to your sensitivity to solanine.

Solution

If you are troubled by stubborn stiffness that does not respond to the usual internal washing and detoxification programs, then you may be allergic to the nightshade group of foods.

Simple Detoxification Plan

Eliminate tomatoes, potatoes, eggplants, and green or red peppers in any form from your food program. These are four high-solanine foods that can lead to pain and arthritic distress. The nightshade foods may cause toxic overload in some people and subsequent arthritis distress. Eliminating them from your diet is a simple detoxification plan that may well banish arthritis reactions.

CASE HISTORY—No-Nightshade Diet-No Arthritis Pain in Eight Days

A victim of osteoarthritis (degenerative joint disease) for ten years, farmer Morton A. faced serious financial losses since he was unable to work his land. The expense of hired hands made it a losing proposition. Medications gave him side effects worse than the stiffness and debilitation of his osteoarthritis. He needed help badly. He received it from a food technologist at the nutrition laboratory connected with the local university hospital. Morton A. was tested, found to be allergic (yes, allergic!) to the nightshade group of foods. Allergic symptoms erupted into osteoarthritis. Morton A.'s joints and muscles had toxic waste overload; cells were encrusted with debris from faulty metabolism of the *solanine* contained in the nightshade foods. This allergy was responsible for the near-crippling arthritis pain.

Morton A. was put on a simple detoxification plan. It called for one simple change: avoid the four nightshade foods listed above in any form. He received his reward within three days. He had increased flexibility of his arms and legs. At the end of the sixth day, he was able to do routine chores with the vitality of a youngster. By the eighth day, he was so energetic and flexible, he released his hired workers and did most of the farming himself. Not only was his farm saved from financial disaster, he himself was saved—from crippling confinement. By avoiding the four nightshade foods, he detoxified his system and was free of arthritis—and became young again!

THE OIL THAT CLEANS AWAY "ARTHRITIS SLUDGE"

Remember the cod liver oil your parents gave you as a youngster throughout the winter to help protect you against colds? Haven't taken it in years? Then rediscover it. Certain types of fish oils may help protect against inflammation flare-ups of rheumatoid arthritis and protect against the sludge destruction of your limbs. Avoiding bad flare-ups may help improve your resistance to arthritis and initiate a washing away of free radicals and hurtful toxic wastes.

Fish Oils to the Rescue

Scientists have discovered that fish oils are able to create a detoxification reaction that will soothe and cool off arthritic inflammation. Fish oil, a polyunsaturated fat, creates this cleansing because it contains Omega-3 fatty acids, not Omega-6 fatty acids, which are abundant in other polyunsaturated fats. Your body turns Omega-6 fatty acids (which are essential to health) into inflammatory chemicals called leukotrienes. But, Omega-3 fatty acids serve as alternative building blocks for biochemical products, and they have far less inflammatory potential.

Omega-3 fatty acids in fish oils produce "good" prostaglandins (hormone-like substances) that do not cause inflammation or pain. In other words, fish oil blocks the cause of inflammation and protects against pain. The Omega-3 fatty acids reduce the body's production of arachidonic acid. This antagonistic acid often causes inflammation of joints and other tissues. The Omega-3 fatty acids in fish oil take the place of the body's normal fatty acids, boost your inner cleansing action, and free your body from the excess of arachidonic acid that is responsible for painful inflammation. With this detoxification reaction, your joints are less tender, your circulation is improved, and your inflammation is cooled.

Unique Cleansing Power

Fish oil contains a unique essential detoxifying fatty acid known as *eicosapentaenoic acid*. This jawbreaker of a substance—EPA for short—is propelled into your blood vessels. Here, EPA becomes an *anti-aggregating* substance, able to break down blood sludge and prepare it for elimination. This unique cleansing power is available in fish oils.

How to Take

Fish containing the highest potency of Omega-3 fatty acids and EPA include (in order of potency): haddock, cod, pollack, Northern pike, sole, tuna (light in water), red snapper, flounder, turbot, rockfish, Pacific halibut, striped bass, ocean perch, whiting, carp, salmon, whitefish, herring, sablefish. *Suggestion:* Include fish at least three to five times per week as part of your meal program. You will be giving your body the needed detoxifying ingredients, Omega-3 fatty acids and EPA among other nutrients, to help wash away toxic wastes and free your joints from sludge. You will help clean away "arthritis sludge" with this miracle oil from the depths of the oceans!

Capsules Are Available

Health stores and pharmaceutical outlets have fish oil capsules available. Take them with the approval of your health practitioner. More is not necessarily better. The cleansing action of the oil may be overdone and blood will not be able to clot in case of a wound. A little fish oil goes a long way. Moderate amounts of a supplement may be included with your program of eating more fish from the preceding list. (Taking several spoonfuls of pure fish oil can have a drawback. Unlike fish oil capsules, pure fish oil contains heavy amounts of vitamins A and D, which can be risky in high doses.)

CASE HISTORY—**"Oiled Joints" Become Flexible Within One Week**

Martha K. grimaced with pain whenever she had to reach a high shelf in her kitchen cupboard. At times, simple vacuuming so twisted her back that she was bedridden for the rest of the day. She complained of "dry" joints. She might have surrendered to inevitable crippling had not an orthomolecular (nutrition-minded) physician diagnosed her problem as blood sludge. He prescribed more fish throughout the week, especially haddock, cod, pollack, and Northern pike. He also told Martha K. to take fish oil capsules regularly. Almost immediately her joints had less inflammation, and swelling was reduced. She could move with greater agility. By the end of one week, she was able to perform household chores with hardly any pain. Her "oiled joints" had made her young again, thanks to the EPA action that washed out the excessive sedimentation from her body. In effect, the EPA action cleansed her joints—oiled them, so to speak—so that she could say goodbye to arthritis.

THE TINY ANCIENT VEGETABLE THAT CONQUERS ARTHRITIS PAIN

For thousands of years, one vegetable has been hailed as a wonder food with miracle healing benefits. Today, this tiny vegetable has the amazing power of washing your body free of toxic overload to help you overcome arthritis. What is it?

Garlic!

A member of the onion family, garlic is unique because it contains antibacterial and antifungal properties that make it a powerful body cleanser. In modern times, garlic has emerged as a cleansing food with power to fight arthritis.

Secret Pain-Ending Power of Garlic

The power of garlic as a pain-killer may be considered "secret" because for many years this knowledge was confined largely within the medical profession, not well known among lay people. So it is with great excitement that the benefits of garlic are now being made available to all. Here they are:

Garlic gives off an unusual type of ultraviolet reaction called *mitogenetic radiation.* These emissions are called *Gurwitch rays* after the European electrobiologist who first reported their pain-killing powers. These same Gurwitch rays are able to dislodge toxic wastes from their encrusted blockages and then prepare them for elimination. This helps stimulate new cell growth and provide an inner cleansing of irritating substances.

Brings Down Inflammation, Soothes Pain

When you consume garlic, your digestive system, through enzyme activity, will extract a substance from the garlic called *allicin.* Your enzymes take this allicin to promote a scrubbing action to cool down the inflammation that is the bane of rheumatoid and other types of arthritis. This same allicin, from garlic, helps soothe pain by washing away the grating sand-like wastes that stubbornly cling to your vital joints, muscles, and related organs. In so doing, garlic, via the allicin action, is able to help you conquer arthritis pain.

Easy Way to Take Garlic

Potency is highest in the garlic bulb itself. Take three cloves, chop them finely, and add to a raw vegetable salad or any sandwich. Add diced garlic to a bowl of soup. Use garlic for any stew, casserole, or baked dish. Chew a garlic clove or two daily. You will feel the cleansing action very swiftly.

What About Garlic Odor?

Basically, chew a garlic clove and follow it with parsley to mask the odor. No need to be a social outcast. Remember this basic fact: the odor occurs only when you take *raw* garlic. There is no odor from *cooked* garlic. *Tip:* Finish garlic by chewing licorice (chemical-free from health store), or chew on a small cinnamon stick, or some cloves. Or else take raw garlic with grated carrot to mask the odor. (All are available at health stores.) You'll sweeten your breath and be socially acceptable as a garlic eater. You'll also become more flexible in your joints and muscles, thanks to garlic's power of detoxification and cleansing.

HOW TO "STEAM CLEAN" YOUR BODY AND WASH AWAY ARTHRITIS PAIN

Hydrotherapy has long been known as an effective, all-natural way to "steam clean" the body, wash out accumulated toxins, and free your body of stubborn joint-muscle pain. Today, it is recognized as an effective way to detoxify your toxic overload and wash out arthritis pain.

How to "Steam Clean" at Home

Fill your bath with water in the temperature range of 96° F. to 103° F. Slowly immerse yourself. Relax for 15 to 20 minutes. Then let the water run out of the tub. Now stand up. Turn on the shower to a comfortably hot stream, gradually making it lukewarm. Stand for five more minutes under the flow. Turn off the shower, towel dry yourself, and relax in bed. *Suggestion:* Try this "steam cleaning" body program twice daily—in the morning (to ease stiffness), then at night before going to sleep (to ease pain and discomfort).

Detoxification Benefits

A leisurely soak at the above temperatures helps open up your billions of skin pores. While you soak, toxic wastes are steamed right out of your body. At the same time, you will have soothed your nerves and relaxed their irritated state by washing away the grating wastes. When you shower, you wash away the removed toxic wastes that cling to your skin. It is a double action (internal and external) cleansing method that will help your joints and muscles to move with better agility.

All-Natural Internal Detoxification Washing

Your body temperature is controlled by a segment of your brain which serves as a thermostat. This internal thermostat remains constant at about 98.6° F. When you soak in a comfortably hot tub, you turn up this internal thermostat. Immediately, perspiration occurs. As you perspire, you are being treated to a detoxification washing process. You are actually cleansing your internal organs! Just 20 minutes in the tub gives you this joint-muscle-cell scrubbing reaction. You will feel sparkling clean. The irritants and free radical wastes that previously caused internal erosion and subsequent pain will be washed out. This is an ancient remedy that is today recognized as an all-natural detoxification process for washing away arthritis pain.

CASE HISTORY—Ends Morning Stiffness With "Steam Clean" Remedy

Morning stiffness was more like morning agony for Nancy R., who found it excruciatingly painful to get out of bed when the shriek of the alarm went off. As an office supervisor, she could jeopardize her job because of lateness. Yet her stiff muscles and curved back made her walk like a puppet, drive like an invalid, work like a disabled person. It took hours to get over the arthritic pain. It was difficult for her to apply her makeup, to work, or to do ordinary tasks. The company physiotherapist suggested she cleanse her body of pain-causing toxins with the "steam clean" bath in the morning and at night. Almost immediately, Nancy R. felt merciful relief. After four days with this easy detoxification remedy she enjoyed restored flexibility to most of her body. By the fifth day, she bounced out of bed with youthful agility and breezed through her activities like a youngster. She was so invigorated, she could work overtime whenever called upon. And she never felt tired! The damaging pain was gone, thanks to her "steam cleaned" and detoxified joints and muscles.

NINE WAYS TO CLEANSE YOUR BODY WITH STRETCHING

Dr. Jack Soltanoff, a leading chiropractor-nutritionist, has found that a set of easy stretching motions help detoxify the system and promote a feeling of youthful flexibility. "Many arthritics are able to move freely and nip the problem in the bud with a total body approach using these stretching remedies '

1. *Standing Reach.* Stand erect with your feet shoulder-width apart and your arms extended over your head. Stretch as high as possible, keeping your heels on the ground. Count slowly to fifteen.

2. *Flexed Leg Back Stretch.* Stand erect with your feet shoulder-width apart and your arms at your sides. Slowly bend over, touching the ground between your feet. Keep your knees relaxed and flexed. Count slowly to fifteen or thirty. If at first you can't reach the floor, touch the top of your shoe line. Repeat two or three times.

3. *Alternate Knee Pull.* Lie on your back with your feet extended and hands at your sides. Pull one leg to your chest, grasp with both arms, and count slowly to five. Repeat seven to ten times with each leg.

4. *Double Knee Pull.* Lie on your back with your feet extended and hands at your sides. Pull both of your legs to your chest. Lock your arms around your legs and pull your buttocks slightly off the ground. Hold and count slowly to twenty or forty. Repeat seven to ten times.

5. *Supine Hip Rotators.* Lie flat on your back with your legs together and your arms away from your sides, palms down. Pull your knees toward your chest and rotate your hips and legs to the left until they are touching the floor. Keep your shoulders and back flat. Repeat, rotating your hips and legs to your right side. Repeat two to four times on each side.

6. *Seated Pike Stretch.* Sit on the floor with your legs extended and your knees together. Exhale and stretch forward slowly, sliding your hands down to your ankles. Try to touch your kneecaps with your chin, keeping your legs as straight as possible. Hold position and count slowly to five or ten. Return to your starting position, inhaling deeply. Repeat four to six times.

7. *The Swan.* Lie on your back, with your arms at your sides, palms down. Bring your knees to your chest while elevating your hips. Bring your legs over your head, trying to touch the floor behind you. As you progress, try to touch your knees to the floor. Hold and count slowly to five or ten. Return to starting position, bending your knees as you lower your legs. Inhale deeply and repeat three to five times.

8. *The Dove.* Stand with your feet apart, legs slightly bent, and your hands clasped behind your back. Slowly bend forward at the waist while elevating your arms behind your back to the "stretching point." Count slowly to five or eight. Relax. Repeat.

9. *Achilles Stretch.* Stand facing a wall, about two feet away. Lean into the wall with your arms extended. Move your left leg forward one-half step, right leg backward one-half step or more. Lower your right heel to the floor. Lower your body toward the wall, stretching the heel tendon in your right leg. Count slowly to five or ten. Reverse leg position. Repeat, performing exercise three to six times on each leg.

Remember: There should be NO pain when stretching. If you feel any discomfort, ease up. Progress slowly through each stretching exercise. Take deep breaths. Relax, if need be, before continuing.[1]

HOW TO WARM UP COLD HANDS OR FEET

Herbs and everyday spices (you probably have them in your kitchen cupboard right now) help revitalize a sluggish circulation to put youthful warmth in your cold limbs. (Some of these detoxifying items are available at health stores or herbal pharmacies.)

- Massage hands and/or feet with warmed macerated oil of honeysuckle flowers (*Lonicera caprifolium*). The herb helps dislodge accumulated sludge and bring an increased flow of blood to the surface of your skin.

- For a foot bath to help wash out hurtful free radicals and rejuvenate circulation of cold feet, use an infusion of 1 tablespoon freshly ground mustard seed to 2 quarts water. Enjoy a 15 or 30 minute soak and feel circulation being boosted as wastes wash out.

- Add cayenne seed powder to warm water (about 2 tablespoons to 2 quarts) and soak your feet for 15 minutes. This is a most powerful stimulant to the circulatory system. It helps wash out debris through the pores and revitalize blood flow to your extremities.

- For a beverage, try rose hip tea as a way of recharging your sluggish circulation. Enjoy field horsetail (*Equisetum arvense*) or buckwheat (*Fagopyrum esculentum*) tea daily to further cleanse and strengthen your smaller capillaries.

- Reduce painful swelling with a drop of undiluted lavender or eucalyptus oil. To soothe any lingering hurt, apply a cold compress of tincture of calendula or calendula ointment.

Pain-Easing Changes to Make Today

Give your body a chance to wash out toxic accumulations and wastes with some better self-care. You'll rid yourself of irritants and help ease pain and enjoy more flexibility with a total body approach—beginning today!

1. *Lose Overweight.* Excess pounds can cause and worsen arthritis. Obesity causes fluctuating hormone levels that lead to distress. Moderate weight is helpful. (Being "pencil thin" is a major risk factor for osteoporosis or bodywide skeletal thinning that can be as disabling as arthritis.) With comfortable weight, you ease stress and pain on your spinal column, knees, hips, ankles, and feet. Lose weight and you wash out stress-causing wastes that hurt your cartilage or otherwise render you vulnerable to inflammation and pain.

2. *Avoid Stress.* Tension increases hurt and causes a buildup of waste products that can worsen arthritic symptoms. Do everything in moderation . . . when you are feeling good. Do a little every day, whether you have a flare-up or not. Follow relaxation techniques such as 30-minute meditation sessions daily.

3. *Morning Stiffness Can Be Soothed.* To ease morning stiffness, apply a muscle ointment at night before going to bed. A herbal rub gives you an emotional boost, too. Next morning, you should be more flexible.

4. *Warm Herbal Rub.* Apply a eucalyptus ointment to the aching part. Rub in gently. The warmth is soothing. Then wrap the aching part in plastic and let the comforting herb seep into your pores, push the waste materials out of your body. Or else, apply a warm towel to the region. After only 30 minutes it is very soothing.

5. *Water Treatment.* In a tub (or a pool at a local health club) try simple walking, bending motions, waving, even jogging. The gentle pressure

against the water's natural resistance and buoyancy helps free your body of congestion.

6. *Cool Off Your Pain.* For an overworked joint, apply ice in a plastic bag or wrap a package of frozen food in a plastic bag and apply for 20 minutes. Remove for 15 minutes. Repeat at least ten times, if needed. It is a form of contrast that will revive a sluggish circulation and help cleanse your joint for better mobility.

7. *Vitamin C Rebuilds Tissues.* About 1000 milligrams of vitamin C daily is helpful. Your cells and tissues have been injured by wastes and sludge and need to be rebuilt with this important vitamin. Also boost your intake of fresh fruits and vegetables for more vitamin C.

8. *Vegetable Oil? Say NO Until You Are Healed.* Granted that polyunsaturated vegetable oil is beneficial but if you are severely hurt by arthritis and taking foods rich in Omega-3 fatty acids, cut back on oil-containing products such as fried foods, margarines, and salad dressings. *Reason:* These foods are rich in Omega-6 fatty acids which could cause inflammation in those who have rheumatoid arthritis. *Tip:* Two oils low in Omega-6 fatty acids are olive oil and canola oil (made from rapeseed). Use these . . . but in moderation. Overall, keep the fat level in your diet at less than 30 percent of total calories.

BIOLOGICAL WASHING: KEY TO ARTHRITIS FREEDOM

Refresh your trillions of cells, your joints, and your muscles with these simple at-home programs. They help initiate vital biological washing that scrubs away pain-causing sediment from your body organs so you can enjoy freedom from arthritis.

—————————— *HIGHLIGHTS* ——————————

1. *Toxic waste overload—a cause of arthritis—needs to be biologically washed out of your system to end this painful problem.*

2. *Edna J. was able to "wash away arthritis" on an easy (and tasty) two-day raw food plan.*

3. *"Hopeless" arthritis can become healed on a nightshade-free program. The simple plan: omit four foods and solve this pain-causing problem.*

4. *Morton A. ended ten years of osteoarthritis in only eight days on a no-nightshade diet.*

5. *Fish oils are able to clean away "arthritis sludge."*

6. *Martha K. conquered crippling pain by following the fish oil program for only one week.*

7. *Garlic is a miracle vegetable with a powerhouse of pain-ending ingredients.*

8. *"Steam clean" your body and end arthritis pain.*

9. *Nancy R. overcame morning stiffness on a simple "steam clean" remedy at home. In minutes, biological washing helped ease distress.*

10. *A doctor recommends a set of nine stretching motions that ease stiffness and boost refreshing circulation.*

11. *Everyday herbs and spices help warm up cold hands or feet.*

12. *Detoxify your body with the set of pain-easing changes you need to make right away. Begin today!*

Chapter 2

THE CHOLESTEROL CLEANSING-WAY TO LONGER LIFE

With the use of everyday foods, you can help clean out cholesterol overload and improve your quality of health so that you have greater protection against arteriosclerosis (hardening of the arteries) and related heart disorders. These miracle foods have the power to loosen, dissolve, and wash out accumulated cholesterol through a dynamic "scrubbing" action. By enjoying more of these foods (and less of others), you will be able to give yourself an around-the-clock, cholesterol-cleansing metabolism, the key to a longer, healthier, and younger lifespan.

CHOLESTEROL—TOXIC SLUDGE

What Is Cholesterol?

Cholesterol is a waxy, fatlike substance found in all animal fats and animal oils, in egg yolks, in dairy products, and in animal foods. In its pure form, it is a tasteless, odorless, white fatty alcohol substance.

Your Body Makes Cholesterol

Cholesterol sludge comes from two sources. It is produced by your liver and is used to make other substances your body needs, such as bile acids and certain hormones. It is also a critical component of all cell membranes. Your liver can manufacture all the cholesterol your body needs.

Cholesterol can also enter your body from your diet. Foods of animal origin, such as meat, poultry, fish, eggs, and cheese and other dairy products, all provide some cholesterol. Your liver takes substances from these foods and puts them through a biological condensation process to create the compound *squalene*, the precursor of cholesterol.

Can You Have Too Much?

You *do* need some cholesterol for the synthesis of bile acids: it is essential for digestion and absorption of fats in your intestine. Your endocrine glands use cholesterol in making valuable steroid hormones. Cholesterol is also present in your central nervous system. When faced with stress or tension, your body sends forth additional cholesterol to meet the challenges of increased nerve response. So, you must have *adequate* cholesterol.

What's the Problem?

When too much cholesterol sludge accumulates in your bloodstream, heart disease can develop. Cholesterol travels through the bloodstream to the body tissues in droplets called *lipoproteins*. There are two types of lipoproteins:

1. *Low density lipoproteins (LDL)*—the "bad" type. When too much LDL accumulates in the bloodstream, the artery walls become filled with sludge, causing the inside of the arteries to narrow. This interferes with the flow of blood and can result in a heart attack.
2. *High density lipoproteins (HDL)*—the "good" type. This type carries cholesterol away from your body tissues back to your liver for disposal.

If excessive cholesterol is allowed to remain and accumulate, it causes internal blockages throughout your body and you run the risk of a stroke, high blood pressure, and heart trouble. Your body weakens. Health starts to decline. The blame: toxic waste overload.

How Much Cholesterol You Need?

The risk of coronary artery disease increases as your blood cholesterol level rises. It is estimated that one out of every two adults have readings of 200 mg/dl (milligrams per deciliter) or greater. This places them at an increased risk of coronary disease.

Your doctor will measure your level with a blood sample taken from your finger or your arm and will confirm the result with a second test if it is greater than 200 mg/dl. The following table shows you how the readings of your total blood cholesterol tests relate to your risk of developing heart problems.

Desirable Blood Cholesterol Under 200 mg/dl	Borderline-High Blood Cholesterol 200 to 239 mg/dl	High Blood Cholesterol Over 240 mg/dl

Note: These categories apply to anyone 20 years of age or older.

A blood cholesterol level of 240 mg/dl or greater is considered "high" blood cholesterol. But any level above 200 mg/dl, even in the "borderline-high" category, increases your risk for heart disease. CAUTION: If your reading is 240 mg/dl or greater, you have more than twice the risk of someone whose reading is 200 mg/dl. You need to take corrective steps right away.

EVERYDAY FOODS THAT SCRUB AWAY STUBBORN CHOLESTEROL SLUDGE

High blood cholesterol can be reversed. The accumulated plaques can be broken down, melted, and washed out of your body. Several power foods are able to create this internal cleansing. Let's see how you can use them to enjoy a longer and younger lifeline.

Garlic Can Unplug Your Arteries

An all-natural waste-scrubber, garlic has the power to break down plaques that have glued themselves inside and outside your arteries. Garlic will protect against the development of atherosclerosis and heart trouble.

Scrubbing Power of Garlic

This miracle waste-scrubbing vegetable contains *allicin,* an active sulfur-containing compound that is digestively transformed into *diallyldisulfide.* This initiates a powerful internal scrubbing action that reduces the lipid (fat) levels in your liver and bloodstream. This same compound works swiftly to break down accumulated fats and prepare them for elimination.

Benjamin Lau, M.D., professor at California's Loma Linda University School of Medicine, where he has taught medical microbiology and immunology, tells us,

"Let's find out how garlic affects high blood lipids. The scientific data we have available demonstrate at least three possibilities. (1) Garlic has been shown to either inhibit or reduce endogenous lipogenesis. (2) Garlic has been shown to increase breakdown of lipids and to enhance elimination of the breakdown by-products through the intestinal tract. (3) Garlic has been shown to move the lipids from the tissue depot to the blood circulation and subsequently to be excreted from the body."

Dr. Lau tells of studies that demonstrate that "components of garlic inhibit lipid synthesis by liver cells." With the use of garlic, preferably on a daily basis, you will promote a scrubbing action that will help control the levels of cholesterol sludge to protect against cardiovascular distress.[2]

Eat Garlic With Each Meal

One or two garlic cloves chewed thoroughly, each day, or chopped and added to your meal (each day) will send forth this powerful allicin into your system to create the vital unplugging of your arteries. Garlic is a dynamically powerful cell-scrubber that uproots and washes out this toxic waste.

CASE HISTORY—A Garlic Clove a Day Keeps Cholesterol Way-Way-Way Down

Paul B. was a heavy construction worker who craved solid but fatty meat meals. He developed a problem—excessively high cholesterol readings of 280 mg/dl. His company doctor prescribed the daily use of garlic along with reduction of fat intake. Paul B. liked the tangy taste of garlic and would consume as many as four cloves either with or at the end of his lunch and dinner. His breakfast was usually light, so it needed no garlic cleanser. In nine days, Paul B.'s cholesterol levels dropped at least 30 milligrams. At the end of fourteen days, it was 220 mg/dl. At the end of twenty-eight days, he had a favorable 190 mg/dl reading. He continued enjoying his favorite foods but with fat reduction and the important garlic "dessert" as he happily and healthfully called it. Only one clove a day was enough to keep his cholesterol at a healthy level.

HOW LECITHIN WASHES AWAY CHOLESTEROL SLUDGE

Lecithin is a bland, water-soluble, granular powder made from de-fatted soybeans. Biochemists call it a *phosphatide,* that is, an essential component of all living cells and tissues. It is a prime source of phosphorus and nitrogen.

How Does It Wash Sludge?

A digestive enzyme, *lecithinase,* takes ingested lecithin and dispatches its choline (a B-complex vitamin) into the bloodstream. This lecithin-released choline is able to break down cholesterol deposits and actually wash them right out of your system. Lecithin also contains lipotropic agents which metabolize the sludge and bring about its elimination.

Special Cleanser. Lecithin contains substances which clear up *vitreous opacities* (a colorless thickening, the forerunner of cholesterol deposits) and wash them out of your cells before they are able to accumulate into sludge.

Breaks Down Fatty Wastes. Lecithin stimulates the distribution of *esterases* (enzyme activators) in the bloodstream, which act swiftly to break down fatty waste accumulations, to clean your arteries.

Double-Action Cell Cleansing. Lecithin is a prime source of two cell cleansers: *phosphatides* and *sitosterols*. They have the unique power of breaking down plaques and washing them out of your system. This gives you double-action cell cleansing that works swiftly and effectively.

CASE HISTORY—**Melts, Eliminates Thick Cholesterol in Twelve Days**

Susan O. was told by her cardiologist that she had unusually high levels of cholesterol. The problem was serious. The wastes were thick and resisted usual nutritional methods of dissolution. Susan O. was advised to take from six to eight tablespoons of lecithin granules daily (available at health stores). She could mix them with vegetable juices, or sprinkle over cereals, salads, in stews, soups, casseroles. Susan O. followed this advice, cutting down on animal and fatty foods, too. Within twelve days, the stubborn cholesterol plaques succumbed to the emulsifying power of the lecithin and actually washed right out of her body. Her cardiologist told her the good news—she had a cholesterol reading of 180 mg/dl, thanks to the lecithin program.

PECTIN FOR BALANCE OF HDL-LDL REACTIONS

Pectin is a water-soluble substance in plant foods that yields a gel used as the basis for jellies. It is a natural cell-scrubber derived mainly from plant cell walls and citrus fruit pulp. Pectin also has the power of being able to balance the delicate HDL-LDL levels in your bloodstream.

HDL Versus LDL

HDL and LDL are two different substances that are poles apart. One causes wastes to accumulate. The other helps scrub them out. Let's see the difference.

1. HDL stands for *high density lipoprotein*, a form of fat circulating in your bloodstream. It is beneficial because it is a cleanser. The more HDLs you have, the cleaner your cells.

2. LDL stands for *low density lipoprotein*, a form of cholesterol sludge that accumulates in your bloodstream. It is hazardous because an excessive accumulation of LDL sludge causes a risk of arterial and coronary ill health.

Problem

In many situations, an excess of LDLs will "overpower" the HDLs. This causes the cells to become filled with fatty wastes, a serious cardiovascular risk.

Why This Conflict?

Because water and fat do not mix, your body needs a method for dislodging excess fatty wastes (including cholesterol) and transporting them via your bloodstream for excretion. Proteins are used for this purpose. Scientists have named the two major groups of cholesterol-protein aggregates HDLs and LDLs.

What's the Difference?

Here is the key to solving this internal struggle. HDLs act like cell-scrubbers, moving throughout your body via your bloodstream, searching out plaques and wastes and removing them from your cells; then the scrubbing HDLs carry these wastes to your liver and other channels for elimination. This is a vital cleansing action.

Danger

Opposing this cleansing action are the LDLs. These act as "delivery trucks" by picking up fats, wastes, cholesterol, toxic clumps, and actually depositing them throughout your cells, especially in your blood vessels.

What's the Problem?

Your general health depends on the balance of this cleansing-removal-delivery system. If you have an excess of LDLs, then your cells become overloaded, overflowing with wastes and refuse.

Answer

Boost your release of the cleansing HDLs so they are able to gather up these wastes and prepare them for elimination.

How Pectin Boosts HDLs, Washes Cells, Creates Balance

You need to boost the vigor of your cell-scrubbing HDLs. Pectin is a food that has this power. When pectin enters your metabolism, it works speedily in boosting levels of HDLs so that they can "attack" cholesterol and waste products and protect against overload. Pectin boosts the vigor of HDLs so they can more effectively wash your cells.

Dynamic Power of Pectin

An indigestible fiber, pectin becomes converted to an acid that combines with cholesterol, tri-glycerides, and wastes to form an insoluble salt. Pectin's goal is to wash out this "package" of debris. Similarly, pectin binds with many of these plaquelike toxic wastes. It blocks their absorption within your cells and both on and in your arteries. Pectin actually seizes these wastes and sends them through your eliminative channels. All this is done by boosting the helpful HDL levels so that the choking LDL levels are overcome.

How to Take Pectin

Be not deceived! Consuming big gobs of jelly is *not* the wise way to take pectin. You'll only fill up on sugar (a non-nutritive flavoring) which comprises up to 75 percent of most jellies. You'll be adding empty calories and leaving yourself open to other ailments caused by sugar, so pass up this idea. Instead, you will find pectin in apples. Whether whole, sliced, grated, or made into applesauce (without sugar or artificial ingredients), you'll have adequate amounts of pectin. Be sure to eat the skin (after washing the fruit, of course) where pectin exists in its highest concentration. *Tip:* One apple has about two grams of pectin. Ten grams daily are helpful in boosting the cell-scrubbing HDL levels to guard against toxic waste overload.

Other sources of pectin include such fresh fruits as bananas, pineapples, cherries, grapes, peaches, raspberries, figs, and sun-dried raisins. Also try tomatoes, avocados, carob, sunflower seeds, and sesame seeds. Plan to eat these foods daily in any desired variety. You'll boost your HDL levels and control the amount of sludge that the undesirable LDLs would otherwise be dumping on your cells.

FIVE EASY WAYS TO BOOST CELL-WASHING ACTIONS

Your goal is to block overreaction of LDLs and to increase the cell-washing function of the HDLs. To do so, you need to establish an internal ratio so that you have more HDLs. Here is a set of ways to boost the cell-washing action and enjoy more youthful health:

1. *Give up smoking.* Smoking knocks out the beneficial HDLs. At the same time, it raises the cell-dirtying LDLs. To guard against this antagonistic reaction, give up smoking. It's good for your total health.

2. *Keep physically active.* Regular exercise boosts your levels of important HDLs. Even regular walking boosts the cell-washing action of the HDLs. CAUTION: A sedentary lifestyle leads to more sludge-depositing LDLs, which in turn increase your risk of cardiovascular disorders. Keep active and you keep your cells clean.

3. *Make dietary adjustments.* Reduce saturated fats—they raise your cholesterol level more than anything else you eat. Use more whole grains, seafood, and vegetables.

4. *Control your weight.* Being overweight may also increase your blood cholesterol levels. With weight reduction, you are able to help bring down the readings and improve the cell-washing process.

5. *The stress connection.* Stress reportedly is able to raise blood cholesterol levels. There may be other explanations for this effect. For example, during times of stress, you have a tendency to eat more foods that are high in saturated fat and cholesterol, which may increase your blood cholesterol levels. By minimizing stress, you may help keep your cholesterol under control.

Less Sludge = Longer Lifeline

Lowering your high blood cholesterol will simultaneously help wash out the fatty buildup in the walls of your arteries and reduce your risk of heart attack and death. In adults with "high" blood cholesterol levels, for each 1 percent reduction in total cholesterol levels, there is a 2 percent reduction in the number of heart attacks. In other words, if you reduce your cholesterol level by 15 percent, your risk of coronary heart disease could be lowered by 30 percent

TEN WAYS TO PROTECT AGAINST CHOLESTEROL OVERLOAD

Make some simple adjustments in your food program. You'll help protect against overloading your cells with cholesterol sludge. Here's a set of suggestions for cleaning your organs—and keeping them clean.

1. Eat no more than three egg yolks a week, including those in cooking. Egg whites are free of cholesterol and so may be eaten freely. (Give the egg yolks to your family pet!)

2. Limit use of organ meats and shellfish.

3. In any planned meat meals for the week use poultry without the skin or fish; limit beef or lamb to three moderate-sized portions per week.

4. Choose lean cuts of meat. Trim away all visible fat. Discard fat that cooks out of the meat.

5. Avoid deep fat frying; use cooking methods that help remove fat: baking, boiling, broiling, roasting, stewing.

6. Restrict (better yet, avoid) use of fatty luncheon and variety meats such as sausages and salami.

7. Instead of butter and other solid or hydrogenated fats, use liquid vegetable oils (in moderation—these are fats, too) that have valuable waste-washing polyunsaturates. A little goes a long way.

8. Instead of whole-milk products, use those made from low-fat or nonfat milk.

9. Egg whites do not contain cholesterol so you can eat them regularly. They also contain lecithin, a powerful sludge-washer, so this can be a power food for your program.

10. Consume at least three or four cloves of garlic daily. This miracle food not only lowers cholesterol, but also washes out the most harmful part of fat—the low density lipoprotein (LDL) fraction. *Bonus:* Garlic reduces the tendency of blood platelets to clump together abnormally because of excessive toxic wastes. Such a clumping can predispose a threatening blood clot (forerunner of stroke, heart attack, or both!). So be sure to wash your cells with the intake of garlic every single day!

What Should Your Blood Cholesterol Goal Be?

A total cholesterol level below 200 mg/dl and an LDL-cholesterol below 130 mg/dl are desirable. To help maintain these readings, plan to consume no more than 300 milligrams of cholesterol daily. *Careful:* One egg yolk gives you close to this limit. One small portion of organ meat may give you more than the limit.

CHOLESTEROL

Elevated blood cholesterol has been identified as one of the major factors associated with an increased risk of developing coronary heart disease.

Cholesterol is an essential fat-like substance found in all body cells. Our bodies manufacture cholesterol out of materials derived from foods we eat.

By lowering the intake of both *dietary cholesterol* and of *saturated fats*, blood cholesterol can be lowered.

Cholesterol is present in animal food products—meats, poultry, fish, eggs, and dairy products containing butter fat. Common foods highest in cholesterol are brains, kidney, sweetbreads, liver, and egg yolk.

Cholesterol is not found in plant foods—fruits, vegetables, grain and cereal products, and nuts.

PRINCIPAL SOURCES OF CHOLESTEROL

Food and Description	Edible Amount	Milligrams Cholesterol
Eggs		
Chicken, whole	1 large	274
Chicken, white only	1 large	0
Duck, whole	1 large	619
Organ Meats		
Brains, beef, calf, pork, lamb	3½-oz. raw	1985
Heart, beef	3½-oz. cooked	274
Heart, chicken	3½-oz. cooked	231
Kidney, beef, calf, pork, lamb	3½-oz. cooked	804
Liver, beef, calf, pork, lamb	3½-oz. cooked	438
Liver, chicken	3½-oz. cooked	746
Sweetbreads	3½-oz. cooked	466
Meat		
Beef, bone removed	3½-oz. cooked	94
Chicken, flesh and skin—breast	3½-oz. cooked	80
Chicken, flesh and skin—drumstick	3½-oz. cooked	91
Lamb, bone removed	3½-oz. cooked	98
Pork, bone removed	3½-oz. cooked	89
Turkey, flesh and skin	3½-oz. cooked	93
Veal, bone removed	3½-oz. cooked	101
Shellfish		
Clams, soft	12 large raw	72
Crabs, steamed in shell	1 cup meat	125
Crabs, canned	½-cup packed	80
Lobster, cooked	1 cup meat	123
Oysters, Eastern	12 raw	90
Shrimp, canned drained solids	½-cup (approx. 12 large)	96
Fish		
Cod, flesh only	3½-oz. raw	50
Cod, dried, salted	3½-oz.	82
Flounder, flesh only	3½-oz. raw	50
Haddock, flesh only	3½-oz. raw	60
Halibut, flesh only	3½-oz. raw	50
Herring, flesh only	3½-oz. raw	85

PRINCIPAL SOURCES OF CHOLESTEROL

Food and Description	Edible Amount	Milligrams Cholesterol
Herring, canned, solids and liquids	3½-oz.	97
Mackerel, flesh only	3½-oz. raw	95
Mackerel, canned, solids and liquids	3½-oz.	95
Roe, salmon	1 oz. raw	101
Salmon, sockeye or red—flesh only	3½-oz. raw	35
Salmon, canned, solids and liquids	3½-oz.	35
Sardines, canned in oil, drained solids	3½-oz.	140
Tuna, canned in oil, drained solids	3½-oz.	65

Fats

Butter, regular	1 Tbsp.	33
Butter, whipped	1 Tbsp.	22
Cream, heavy	1 Tbsp.	21
Cream, light	1 Tbsp.	10
Cream, half and half	1 Tbsp.	6
Cream, sour	1 Tbsp.	5
Lard	1 Tbsp.	13
Margarine, all vegetable fat	1 Tbsp.	0
Mayonnaise	1 Tbsp.	10

Milk and Milk Products

Cheese, cheddar	1 oz.	30
Cheese, processed American	1 oz.	27
Cheese, cottage, creamed	½-cup	16
Cheese, cottage, low fat (2% fat)	½-cup	10
Cheese, cream	1 oz.	31
Cheese, ricotta, whole milk	½-cup	63
Cheese, ricotta, partially skim milk	½-cup	38
Ice Cream, regular (approx. 10% fat)	1 cup	59
Ice Cream, rich (approx. 16% fat)	1 cup	88
Ice Cream, French, soft serve	1 cup	153
Ice Cream, frozen custard	1 cup	97
Ice Milk, hardened	1 cup	18
Ice Milk, soft serve	1 cup	13
Milk, whole	1 cup	33
Milk, low fat, 2% fat	1 cup	19
Milk, low fat, 1% fat	1 cup	10
Milk, nonfat (skim)	1 cup	5
Milk, chocolate flavored milk	1 cup	30
Milk, buttermilk, cultured	1 cup	9
Yogurt, whole milk, plain	1 cup	29
Yogurt, lowfat, plain	1 cup	14
Yogurt, lowfat, fruit varieties	1 cup	12
Yogurt, skim milk, plain	1 cup	4

YOUR CHOLESTEROL-WATCHING CHART

As previously explained, cholesterol is made by your body and also is found in foods. So you need to control intake of this sludge because of the risk of an excess. Limit yourself to 300 milligrams—even a bit less—daily, and you should be on safe ground.

On pages 24–25 is a chart listing common foods and their cholesterol content. Plan your meals with proper levels in mind daily. You'll help keep your body clean and make it easier for the power foods to control HDL-LDL levels, the key to internal washing.

HOW FIBER SWEEPS CHOLESTEROL OUT OF YOUR BODY

Fiber is a substance in your diet that is not digested and provides no nutrients. Yet fiber is a powerful cell-washer and may well be the most important remedy in reducing and cleaning out cholesterol. There are two types of fiber, and you need to know the differences between them.

Insoluble Fiber

This fiber provides bulk which helps in the movement of food and water through your intestines. Insoluble fiber absorbs water, helps soften stool, and reduces the time it takes digested food to move through the bowels. Insoluble fiber is linked to lower rates of colon cancer. It is found in wheat, corn, vegetables, and rice bran products. Lettuce and cauliflower are good sources, too.

Soluble Fiber

This fiber helps rid your body of bile acids, metabolites synthesized from body cholesterol. A steady intake of foods containing soluble fiber affects your body's own production of LDL cholesterol—the "bad" cholesterol that clogs arteries and leads to increased risk for heart attacks. It is found in dried beans, carrots, oranges, bananas and other fruits, and most grains. Good sources are foods made from whole grain barley, whole grain oats, and oat bran.

LOWER CHOLESTEROL WITH ONE CUP OF CLEANSING FOODS A DAY

Oat bran and dried beans are powerful cleansing foods that can lower your cholesterol almost at once—and all you need is one cup per day.

James W. Anderson, M.D., of the University of Kentucky, Lexington has found that men with high cholesterol levels who ate 100 grams a day of oat bran (about two servings of oat bran hot cereal) reduced their total blood cholesterol levels by 27 percent in only seven to eleven days. A 19 percent cholesterol reduction was sustained through the end of the twenty-eight-day study.

Oat Bran Is Cleansing Food

Dr. Anderson tells of a study concerning men with high (over 260 mg/dl) cholesterol. When the men were put on a standard diet, but also given oat bran, there was a significant drop in both total cholesterol and the harmful LDL. It did not significantly affect HDL, which helps wash out cholesterol. The men consumed only 100 grams of the oat bran daily to have this cell-washing reaction.

Dried Beans Lower Cholesterol

Eating 100 grams (about one cup) of dried beans a day was found to significantly decrease both total cholesterol and harmful LDL. The beans did lower the important HDL, but the amount was "not statistically significant." (The beans were cooked, obviously.)[3]

Why Oat Bran Is a Vital Cholesterol-Washing Food

Oat bran contains beta-glucan, a powerful ingredient that helps flush out cholesterol when used as part of a fat-modified diet. Oat bran cereals contain more bran—the outer covering of the grain—than do standard oatmeals, which are made from the whole oat grain. (Standard oatmeal has about two-thirds the amount of soluble fiber found in oat bran.)

Two-Step Cholesterol-Washing Plan

Even on a fat-controlled program, cholesterol may still cling stubbornly in excessive amounts. Wash out the sludge with this simple two step plan:

1. Daily, plan to have one cup of oat bran hot cereal. Include different fresh fruit slices to vary the taste from day to day. Add a bit of honey and some non-fat milk for a tasty cholesterol-washing food.
2. Several times a week, include at least one cup of freshly cooked beans as part of a main meal. Even as part of a large raw salad, you will be helping your body set off the metabolism that will wash out excessive cholesterol and control the LDL levels that can threaten your health.

TWO OAT BRAN MUFFINS A DAY KEEP CHOLESTEROL UNDER CONTROL

Oat bran packs a wallop in dislodging cholesterol and washing the sludge out of your cells. Judith S. Stern, Sc.D., of the University of California-Davis has found that "the beta-glucans in oats are water soluble and have a scrubbing effect on lipid (fat) metabolism. Oat bran is one of the few types of fiber that can lower the 'bad' LDL and raise the 'good' HDL. Oats also contain a unique type of protein—much more than other grains—that further promote this cholesterol-washing action." Dr. Stern explains that the soluble fibers found in grain are also beneficial in the slow absorption of glucose which provides more body energy. In the gastrointestinal tract, the oat bran's soluble fiber "enhances elimination of bile acids, resulting in bacterial metabolites which decrease your body's production of cholesterol."

Dr. Stern suggests eating about two oat bran muffins daily—a standard recipe should use an adequate amount of old-fashioned or whole oats—to decrease blood cholesterol. When used with a low-fat program, you will soon have control over cholesterol levels in your body.[4]

Tip: While groats, rolled oats, and steel-cut oats are fine, oat bran seems to be favored. The latter is a finely ground flour product made from the outer seed casing (bran) of the oat groat. Pure oat bran seems to be best for washing out cholesterol, but you may vary it with other oat products to satisfy your taste buds. Try these methods for using oats and oat bran:

- Substitute oat bran for up to one third of the flour in baked goods or as breading for oven-fried fish.
- For a dinnertime side dish, add up to two tablespoons of regular oats to two cups of brown rice.
- For a snack, toast rolled oats with a little oil and cinnamon in a 350° F. oven. Serve as a topping for low- or no-fat yogurt.
- Use 1/3 cup of oats instead of bread crumbs in vegetable loaves or meatballs for every one pound of ground meat. You'll never taste the reduced meat!

Oats: Your Magic Bullet

It is important to include oats and oat bran in your low-fat diet. It lowers LDL and becomes a magic bullet to protect against cholesterol overload.

THE VITAMIN THAT BRINGS DOWN CHOLESTEROL

Niacin, also known as vitamin B₃ does more than lower cholesterol—it washes this dangerous sludge right out of your body. It lowers both total cholesterol and the LDL levels. This cleanser dispatches oxygen to your billions of body cells which then works to free them of accumulated deposits. Niacin also corrects the problem of *sludging*—the bunching up of red cells that might otherwise create a microscopic traffic jam. Niacin liberates these jammed-up cells and creates a washing out of clinging cholesterol.

Food sources include most meats, roasted peanuts, and seafood. Because these foods may have too much fat, cholesterol, or both you may want to try supplements. The U.S. Recommended Daily Allowance is about 20 milligrams. For cholesterol washing, this may be too little. If you are considering a niacin supplement, you will need guidelines.

Kenneth Cooper, M.D., famed cardiologist of Dallas, Texas, has these suggestions: "Large doses of niacin (also known as nicotinic acid) may lower both total cholesterol and LDL cholesterol. It's best to start off with low doses, say up to 100 milligrams a day. Then increase gradually over a period of several weeks to 1000 to 2000 milligrams, three times a day, for a total of 3000 to 6000 milligrams daily."

Dr. Cooper cautions, "Be aware that sudden drastic increases in niacin can produce severe overall flushing, intestinal disorders, and sometimes abnormal liver functions. Be sure to discuss this treatment with your doctor. Niacinamide, a form of niacin that doesn't cause flushing, has no significant effect on blood fats." So the effective cholesterol-washer is niacin, to be used gradually and with your doctor's approval.[5]

──────────────── *HIGHLIGHTS* ────────────────

1. *Cholesterol overload equals internal sludge. Control its intake and be rewarded with a more vigorous and youthful body and mind.*

2. *Paul B. used a few garlic cloves daily to "unplug" his sludge-covered arteries. Garlic acted as a miracle food in cleansing his body.*

3. *Susan O. was able to melt and eliminate thick clumps of cholesterol with the use of an all-natural food, lecithin. It worked cleansing wonders within twelve days.*

4. *Pectin, a natural substance found in many fruits and vegetables, will help balance your HDL-LDL levels.*

5. *Boost cell washing with five easy lifestyle changes.*

6. *Protect against cholesterol overload with ten basic adjustments in your daily living practices.*

7. *Plan your meals with the use of the cholesterol chart. Limit yourself to 300 milligrams daily.*

8. *Fiber—whether in oat bran or in beans—will sweep cholesterol out of your body.*

9. *Niacin (vitamin B_3) is a natural way of helping to detoxify your body on a cholesterol-cleansing program.*

Chapter 3

"FOREVER YOUNG" SKIN THROUGH CATALYTIC CLEANSING

Your skin's ability to look and feel fresh is set back daily. Enemies abound, constantly hampering your efforts to have youthful skin. Pollution is one of these threats. Fumes, exhaust, gases, chemicals, and dirt all take their toll on your skin whether you live in the hub of the city or the rural countryside. Smoking (your own or sidestream) slows up circulation and dulls skin tone. Harsh soaps containing detergents and chemicals can strip away the natural substances that trap moisture, leaving your skin susceptible to aging. Winter air is low in humidity and can dry your skin. What's more, the dry heat you use indoors for warmth and the hot showers you take cause the same skin-aging damage. Perspiration resulting from over-activity can get below your skin's surface and cause intense itching at the elbows, knees, and neck. And of course, the summer sun is damaging, too.

You Can Resist These Skin Threats

You can smooth out wrinkles, clear up blemishes, and restore the glow of youth to your skin. Often, this rejuvenating fresh-faced look can be yours within a few days. Through the simple method of catalytic cleansing, you get to the root cause of your so-called "aging" skin—namely, toxic wastes that have penetrated because of the invasion of the enemies described above. Accumulated, they block the free passage of nutrients causing a "choked" stagnation seen in the form of deep furrows and stubborn blemishes. To better understand how simple home programs can give you a "forever young" skin, let's look at the problem and the internal washing solution.

PROBLEM—SKIN-AGING CELLULITE

What Is It?

Cellulite is a term coined in European health spas to describe those unsightly deposits most visible on thighs and buttocks. Pronounced "cell-uleet," these "hard-to-budge pudge" bulges also accumulate just beneath the skin in the upper arms, back of the neck, shoulders, throat, and face.

What Does It Look Like?

Cellulite is composed of lumpy deposits that resemble chicken skin or a puckery orange skin. Often, it is called the "orange rind" problem. You can *see* cellulite in the form of unattractive bulges, wrinkles, and creases as well as blemishes and discolorations.

What Is the Cause?

Certain body cells have the capacity to store huge amounts of fat; about half of your body's fat is deposited in these cells immediately beneath your skin. Strands of fibrous tissues connect the skin to deeper tissue layers, and also separate the fat cell compartments. When the fat cells increase in size, this causes the compartments of fat to bulge and produces a "waffled" appearance in your skin, similar to the pattern of irregularities on the surface of an orange. *Quick Self-Test:* Compress a skin fold lightly between your fingers. See those imperfections? That's the penalty of cellulite.

Is Waste Accumulation a Factor?

Waste accumulation is the major factor in the development of disfiguring cellulite, a consequence of "fat-gone-wrong." In other words, a combination of fat, water, and toxic wastes that ordinarily should be eliminated from your body stubbornly remains and accumulates.

Why Is This Fat-Waste Sludge Difficult to Remove?

Unlike other sludge accumulations, these wastes gather in the connective tissues that hold fat cells just beneath your skin's surface. Here, round fat-cell chambers are found, along with thin epidermis and corium (thick layer of living tissue), which become thinner and less elastic after the age of thirty. These connective tissues harden and combine with the fat and water. There soon form pockets of a gel-like substance—cellulite. A stubborn substance, it defies ordinary waste removal efforts and starts skin aging that worsens as the years go by.

How Is Cellulite More Resistant Than Ordinary Fatty Deposits?

Cellulite contains more water and waste than ordinary fatty tissue. The big problem is that gel-like cellulite tissue is *stagnant.* Locked, or worse, *trapped* in the cell chambers and the hardening epidermis-corium layers, the wastes cause unsightly bulges and skin blemishes, resisting ordinary waste removal methods.

What Is the Biological Reason for Cellulite Formation?

The connective tissues and fat cells accumulate wastes because of sluggishness by your circulatory system and your liver, which cannot adequately filter toxins out of the cells. When you reach your thirties, there is a slight slowdown of your metabolism. A reduction of the enzymatic cleansing method permits wastes to cling together, to form this unsightly aging condition. It may be considered a "penalty" of going into your middle years.

What Can Be Done to Improve Waste Removal Methods?

A set of home programs will revitalize your sluggish metabolism. These programs will activate your glands and organs to promote more effective removal of wastes. In many situations, the internal (and external) washing methods are so effective, you can see results in a healthier skin in a matter of days, sometimes overnight.

FREE YOUR BODY OF CELLULITE IN FIVE STEPS

Your goal is to dislodge the wastes that have formed a gelatin-like hardness in your connective tissues. Set off an internal washing reaction with this simple five-step cellulite-cleansing program right in your own home.

1. *Foods That Fight Cellulite.* Daily, boost your intake of fresh fruits and vegetables, whole-grain foods, non-fat dairy products, and lots of fresh juices. *Avoid:* sugar, salt, caffeine, artificial foods, chemicals in foods, synthetics, preservatives, additives, and fatty foods—including meat.

   Catalytic Cleansing Benefit: Powerful enzymes found in raw fresh foods will work vigorously to dislodge and break up the clumps of fat-waste accumulations. These enzymes initiate a catalytic cleansing reaction that propels cellulite wastes right out of your eliminative channels. *Special Reward:* By eliminating the items listed under "avoid," you free your body from the onslaught of more wastes. This makes the catalytic removal of wastes all the easier and swifter.

2. *Clean Insides = Youthful Outsides.* Establish regularity by eating high-roughage foods such as wheat germ, bran, whole grains, legumes, fresh fruits, and vegetables daily. Once you are "regular," your

wastes are removed all the more speedily. This is a simple way of washing your overclogged cells and tissues.

Catalytic Cleansing Benefit: Cellulite is an internal clogging problem. Therefore, when you consume these high-roughage, high-fiber foods you stimulate your sluggish metabolism into more vigorous action. Elimination becomes more complete. You remove cellular wastes and help overcome the problem of those unsightly bulges.

3. *Breathe Away Toxic Wastes.* Your choked cells need oxygen. Deprived of this "breath of life," they tend to weaken. Clinging together, they harden because they lack nutrients that are ordinarily transported via the oxygenation process. Without the free exchange of oxygen and carbon dioxide, the cells "choke" and become stagnant. They accumulate wastes and the cellulite syndrome develops. Daily, deep-breathe your way to cellular washing. In the open air or before an open window (avoid drafts or chills) stand and inhale deeply; hold your breath for the count of five. Exhale all the way. Repeat ten to fifteen times each morning. Repeat at night.

   Catalytic Cleansing Benefit: The gentle, forceful intake of oxygen will transport needed nutrients to your waste-burdened cells and tissues. Invigorated, your cells now begin the metabolic process of uprooting and casting out toxic wastes. Give your cells the "breath of life." Clean them through simple inhalation exercises daily. Send fresh circulation streaming through your body. Oxygen-cleansed cells are cellulite-free cells.

4. *Massage Away Those Unsightly Bulges.* A rejuvenating rub is possible with the use of a loofah "sponge," available at most health stores, pharmacies, and beauty supply outlets. The loofah (it grows like a gourd) is a member of the cucumber family. It is fibrous—more than an ordinary massage item. Thousands of these little "needles" rubbed over the bulgy area will dislodge wastes and prepare them for elimination. Use the loofah wet or dry. Loofahs are also available as a hand mitt for easy self-rubbing. Just rub all over your body for about 20 minutes daily, preferably after a bath, and you will soon be rewarded with a smoother skin.

   Catalytic Cleansing Benefit: A loofah will cleanse and stimulate your skin surface. The steady friction penetrates deeper into the lower skin layer and tends to break down and eventually disintegrate accumulated fats and wastes. Stroke the area briskly (but not roughly) in the direction of your heart. Performed daily, you promote a rhythmic removal of age-causing cellulite wastes.

5. *Keep Your Body in Tiptop Shape.* Tension, unrelieved stress, and pent-up emotions are often responsible for waste buildup. The cause is traced to a "choked-up" emotional-physical crisis. This tightness is reflected in clumped-up wastes that lead to skin problems and related disorders. *Example:* You can feel the penalties of tension when you are under so much stress that you become constipated! This suggests you need a change in lifestyle. Plan to have more recreation. Whenever possible, avoid disputes. Shield yourself from excessive responsibilities. Take frequent rest breaks. Relax yourself. In so doing, you revive your body's ability to wash away locked-up wastes.

Catalytic Cleansing Benefit: Loosened-up muscles will help release "kinks" in your arteries, veins, circulatory system, and vital organs. Once these channels are opened up, there is a freer exchange of oxygen and nutrients. Catalytic hormones are able to bring about a more effective dissolution of stubborn clumps and then eject them from your body. By "unlocking" your tension-caused blockages, you rid yourself of unsightly cellulite.

Works Swiftly, Effectively, Permanently, Too. The preceding easy-to-follow five-step cellulite-washing program works quickly. The steps are effective in reviving your metabolism so that you may be permanently rid of cellulite, the cause of aging skin.

CASE HISTORY—Becomes "Forever Young" in One Weekend

Joyce N. was so embarrassed by her wrinkled, furrowed skin she wore long-sleeved garments, high-necked dresses, and wide-brimmed hats to cover her puckered forehead. Costly cosmetics only disguised the problem, which was diagnosed as cellulite by a dermatologist. Joyce N. was told she could stimulate her circulation and wash out the cellulite with the preceding five-step program. It would revive her sluggish metabolism and create a catalytic action that would dislodge and eliminate stubborn fats and wastes. Joyce N. followed the program over a long weekend. Within three days, her wrinkles "ironed out." Her furrows smoothed. Her entire skin was silky soft and rose-colored again. She smilingly boasted she had become "forever young" with only one weekend on this five-step program.

CATALYTIC SKIN CLEANSERS FOR COMMON AND UNCOMMON DISORDERS

Cleanse away skin disorders with these at-home programs, aimed at opening pores, creating a catalytic cleansing action, and rejuvenating your cells so that they become firm, youthful, healthy. Many of these programs work after one or two applications; some require a bit more time. Proceed at your own pace. You have nothing to lose . . . except your aging, blemished skin!

Acne. Apply thin slices of fresh cucumber on acne-plagued areas for 15 minutes. Remove slices. Splash with cold water. Pat dry. Repeat three times daily.

Dry Complexion. Wash your face with a mild soap and warm water. Separate an egg and beat the yolk. Apply to your face. Let yolk harden. After 20 minutes, splash off with warm and cool water. Repeat several times daily. (Remember to keep egg white for use in cooking.)

Oily Complexion. With fingertips, apply plain yogurt to oily areas. Let yogurt remain for 20 minutes. Splash off with tepid water. Repeat several times daily.

Tired Skin. In your palm, combine oatmeal with enough water to make a grainy paste. Gently rub your face with this grainy mixture until dry skin flakes off. Finish with a cold water splash.

Neck Wrinkles. Dip a clean face towel in warm olive oil. Wrap towel around your throat. Cover with a dry towel. After 30 minutes, remove towels and shower off any oil residue. This helps moisturize your neck, steam away toxic wastes, and protect against wrinkles.

Puffy Eyes. Dip cotton balls in milk; apply to your closed eyes. Lie down for 20 minutes. Remove pads and splash with cool water.

Pineapple Skin Cleanser. Into 1/4 cup pineapple juice, dip thick gauze and apply gently to blemished areas of your skin. Let juice remain for 20 minutes, then rinse with tepid water. Repeat twice daily. *Benefit:* Pineapple enzymes help remove the top layer of dead skin cells; pineapple bromelain improves tissue regeneration.

Grape Juice Rinse. Dip clean gauze into a bowl of grape juice. Rub all over your face. Let remain for five minutes. Rinse with tepid and cool water. *Benefits:* The tart elements of the grape juice penetrate skin pores and promote cleansing with cellular regeneration.

Watermelon Pack. Blenderize and strain pitted watermelon chunks. Wrap the pulp in cheesecloth to form a facial pack. Apply this pack to your face. Let remain for 20 minutes. Splash off with cool water. Repeat several times daily. *Benefits:* Nutrients and enzymes in the pack cleanse your pores and introduce much-needed moisture. Watermelon juice helps quench "thirsty" cells beneath the skin surface and protects against wrinkles.

Berry Mask. Wash and hull a handfull of strawberries. Mash with a wooden spoon until smooth. Apply berry mixture to blemishes. Let dry for 20 minutes, then splash off with tepid water. *Benefits:* The high enzyme content catalyzes toxic wastes, initiates cleansing, and creates a glowing skin.

Peachy Complexion. Pit and blenderize several ripe peaches. Smooth on your face as you would a skin cream; it is preferable to leave on overnight. *Benefits:* Peach minerals seep through delicate pores and membranes to promote internal washing so you have more youthful skin.

Dry Skin. Try a moisturizing or home hydrotherapy treatment. Fill tub with warm, *not* hot water (which is drying to the skin). Add one-half cup of ordinary vegetable oil. Soak comfortably while gently washing your face and body with a soft cloth for no more than 15 minutes. Dry with a soft towel, but do not rub. Remember, dry skin is delicate, so treat it with kindness and it will moisturize all the better.

Deep Lines, Creases. Give yourself a gentle massage. Dip fingertips into vegetable oil. Gently massage into the dry portions of your face, always *away* from the direction in which lines tend to form. *Suggestion:* Use an up-and-away motion. Begin at the base of your throat, then work upward and finish at your temples. Let the thin film of oil remain overnight to further moisturize and cleanse while you sleep. Next morning, splash off with warm and cool water. After a few days, your skin will start to smooth out.

Aging Furrows. Mix one handful of raw oatmeal with enough hot mineral water to form a paste; spread onto your face and throat. After it has dried, let remain on your face for 30 minutes. Rinse with cool mineral water. Your creases and wrinkles just "melt" away.

Blackheads, Pitted Dirt. Combine a teaspoon of almond meal (from health store) with enough mineral water; rub this mixture gently into your skin with fingertips. Let dry. Splash off with cool water. Used daily, it helps clear up blackheads and smooths out pitted, dirt-filled pores.

Pore Cleanser and Refiner. Add a pinch of powdered alum (from health store or pharmacy) to enough hot water to form a thin solution. Pat on unsightly pores. When dry, splash off with cool water. This cleanses and tightens enlarged pores, helping to rejuvenate skin.

Total Body Cleanser. Add some dry milk to your bathwater. Soak yourself in this milk bath. Luxuriate for 30 minutes. You'll emerge with a clean body that looks and feels younger than ever.

Rub Away Those Blemishes. Try peels of citrus fruits on blemishes. Orange rind is a helpful complexion softener and facial massage. Grapefruit or lemon peel rubs away chapped blemishes. Rub on affected area gently, as often as possible. Blemishes will begin to clear up almost from the start.

Flaking Skin. Combine one tomato with enough buttermilk to make a smooth paste. Spread over your face, rubbing gently. Let remain for 30 minutes. Splash off with warm and cool water. Wastes and decaying cells are sloughed off. You'll emerge with smoother skin.

Enlarged Pores. Beat one egg white with one teaspoon of lemon juice until stiff. Apply to enlarged pores and blemishes. Let remain for 30 minutes. Wash off with cool water. Pores start to tighten almost at once.

Overnight Skin Cleanser. Combine one tablespoon butter, two tablespoons honey, and one egg yolk. Blend until creamy. Apply to face overnight. It works with catalytic cleansing action *while you sleep.* Next morning, splash off with warm and cool water. Discover a brand new and youthful face smiling happily at you in the mirror.

Steam Away Blemishes. Fill a washbowl with hot water. Toss in a handful of your favorite herbs. Now cover your head with a cloth, making a tent. Steam open your pores for 20 to 30 minutes. The herbal scents penetrate your open pores and initiate a fragrant cleansing. Now, just splash off with cool water to close pores. Blemishes will be cleansed away after a few home steam treatments.

HOW TO RESTORE THE BLOOM OF YOUTH TO YOUR SKIN

"The fundamental influence on how you look and how you age is genetic, but this is very much affected by environmental influences," says Karen Burke, M.D., a New York-based dermatologist whose special interest lies in developing anti-aging techniques. She offers these youth-preserving programs to help you look younger longer:

Avoid abuse to your body. Be especially diligent about avoiding sun exposure without a protective block on your face, hands, and neck. Avoid cold and wind exposure unless you have protective creams. Temper artificially heated environments at home or office with humidifiers.

Maintain your body's natural equilibrium. Weight loss or weight swings from binges followed by crash diets can cause *stria* (stripes) on the skin due to loss of elasticity; weight loss can cause wrinkles in your face. Avoid extremes! No crash diets!

You need some fatty acids for good skin. Include a tablespoon of vegetable oil with your meal program, three times a week. Polyunsaturated fats in moderation will also help plump up your skin.

Water is vital for skin youth. About 70 percent of your skin is water. If you pinch your skin and it doesn't come back quickly, it indicates serious dehydration. You need extra-cellular water in your skin. Water also helps nutrient absorption, fat drainage, and digestion. Drink at least eight 8-ounce glasses of water every single day.

Cleansing rejuvenates your skin. Eliminate harsh alkaline detergents which denature your skin and cause water loss. Use a beauty bar with moisturizing cream. "For more troubled skin," says Dr. Burke, "I recommend using a mild exfoliation technique because it takes off some of the skin layers, helps smooth out wrinkles. Its effect is like lightly sanding a piece of wood, only in this instance, you're gently smoothing the skin's surface each day."

Be cautious of weather assault. Winter is bad for your skin. The extreme cold sends an increased blood flow to the surface to keep your skin warm . . . but this causes more evaporation of water and drier skin. Also indoor heat is very drying and aging to your skin. Humidifiers are essential to counter dry indoor temperatures. We all envy the healthy glow of English and Irish complexions because of the high humidity in those countries. Washing less frequently is a good idea. Use a mild cleanser with moisturizing cream (read label) to remove the extra toxic wastes and dirt.

Do you retain water? Sleep with several pillows to elevate your head. This prevents puffiness in the undereye area when you awaken.

Adjust sleeping position. If you sleep on your stomach or in a prenatal position, you could develop wrinkles on one side of your face. Sleeping face up on your back can help control wrinkles. If this is a difficult position, then make it easier by putting a pillow under your knees.

Which pillow cover to use? A satin pillow cover helps prevent wrinkles. Your skin doesn't stick as much to satin as to cotton or dacron. Polyester fibers should be avoided because they cause excess sweating and sticking.[6]

Water, Moisture, Skin Youthfulness

Water is your skin's cleansing moisturizer. Water keeps your skin pliable. You can maintain youthfulness with this cleansing-rejuvenation remedy:

After you shower or bathe, do not completely towel dry, especially in winter when your skin is driest. Instead, trap the moisture on your skin by applying a moisturizer. Use a dry-skin cream. It prevents water on your skin from evaporating. Moisturizers become the key to a softer skin. Caution: Avoid very hot water. The natural moisturizing substances found in your skin are damaged by very hot water. Instead, use warm or cool water when you wash, then apply a moisturizer while your skin is still damp to preserve softness.

PROTECT YOUR SKIN FROM SUN ABUSE

"Exposure to ultraviolet (UV) radiation, whether from sunlight or tanning parlors, damages your skin; this is a major factor responsible for the increasing number of skin cancers, too," says Douglas David Altchek, M.D., assistant clinical professor of dermatology with Mount Sinai School of Medicine in New York.

Dr. Altchek offers these skin-saving suggestions:

- Use a sunscreen when out in the open, even if it is wintertime.
- Protect your lips with a sunscreen lipstick. Lips are defenseless against sun damage because they contain no protective melanin. Saliva actually magnifies UV radiation.
- Drink plenty of water (eight to ten glasses a day). Your face is the first place to show dehydration.
- Pack plenty of comfortable clothes that will cover your face and other sensitive areas if taking a vacation. Tightly woven cotton is more effective in blocking UV rays than loosely woven synthetics. When skiing or hiking in extremely cold climates, wear a knitted neck cover. While lounging around the pool, it helps to wear a big floppy hat.[7]

Sunscreens Can Save Your Skin

Sunscreens are products designed to help protect your skin. Products carry an SPF designation. What does this mean?

SPF stands for *s*un *p*rotection *f*actor. The amount of time it takes to cause redness or burn is measured by the minimum erythema dose (MED). If it takes one hour of sun exposure to turn you red, and you apply a sunscreen with a SPF of 4, then it will take 4 hours to achieve the same redness. (SPF 4 × 1 hour = 4 hours.) If you apply a SPF of 15, then it will take 15 hours. Remember, everyone is different. If you are fair, blue-eyed, and blonde, then your MED may only be 15 minutes. If you are olive complected, dark-eyed, and have dark hair, then your MED may be 2 hours. Therefore, your protection from a SPF varies.

How Do Sunscreens Protect?

Sunscreens contain chemical ingredients which actually absorb harmful rays of the sun. When applied to your skin, they offer you protection against the abrasive and age-causing assault by the sun. You still need to follow guidelines in saving your skin. Even with SPF products, you may not throw caution to the winds. Far from it!

SIMPLE GUIDELINES TO HELP PROTECT YOU FROM THE DAMAGING RAYS OF THE SUN[8]

1. *Minimize sun exposure* during the hours of 10 a.m. to 2 p.m. (11 a.m. to 3 p.m. daylight saving time) when the sun is strongest. Try to plan your outdoor activities for the early morning or late afternoon.

2. *Wear a hat,* long-sleeved shirts and long pants when out in the sun. Choose tightly-woven materials for greater protection from the sun's rays.

3. *Apply a sunscreen* before every exposure to the sun, and reapply frequently and liberally, at least every two hours, as long as you stay in the sun. The sunscreen should always be reapplied after swimming or perspiring heavily, since products differ in their degrees of water resistance. We recommend sunscreens with an SPF (sun protection factor) of 15 or more printed on the label.

4. *Use a sunscreen* during high altitude activities such as mountain climbing and skiing. At high altitudes, where there is less atmosphere to absorb the sun's rays, your risk of burning is greater. The sun also is stronger near the equator where the sun's rays strike the earth most directly.

5. *Don't forget to use your sunscreen* on overcast days. The sun's rays are as damaging to your skin on cloudy, hazy days as they are on sunny days.

6. *Individuals at high risk for skin cancer* (outdoor workers, fair-skinned individuals, and persons who have already had skin cancer) should apply sunscreens daily.

7. *Photosensitivity*—an increased sensitivity to sun exposure—is a possible side effect of certain medications, drugs and cosmetics, and of birth control pills. Consult your physician or pharmacist before going out in the sun if you're using any such products. You may need to take extra precautions.

8. *If you develop an allergic reaction* to your sunscreen, change sunscreens. One of the many products on the market today should be right for you.

9. *Beware of reflective surfaces!* Sand, snow, concrete and water can reflect more than half the sun's rays onto your skin. Sitting in the shade does not guarantee protection from sunburn.

10. *Avoid tanning parlors.* The UV light emitted by tanning booths causes sunburn and premature aging, and increases your risk of developing skin cancer.

11. *Keep young infants out of the sun.* Begin using sunscreens on children at six months of age, and then allow sun exposure with moderation.

12. *Teach children sun protection early.* Sun damage occurs with each unprotected sun exposure and accumulates over the course of a lifetime.

Courtesy: Skin Cancer Foundation

VITAMINS THAT ACT AS SUNSCREENS

Certain vitamins will help protect your skin from ultraviolet (UV) damage from the inside out—and when applied directly to the skin, says Madhu A. Pathak, Ph.D., senior associate in dermatology and research professor at Harvard Medical School.

Oral Sunscreens

"Vitamins C and E and beta-carotene, the plant-derived precursor of vitamin A, are actually 'oral sunscreens' for your skin," says Dr. Pathak. "These vitamins are powerful antioxidants that act as selective scavengers of 'free radicals'—dangerously reactive oxygen molecules that are generated by many normal biochemical reactions but also by UV light in human skin."

Inner Cleansing Benefit

When taken internally, says Dr. Pathak, the antioxidant vitamins minimize or inhibit the key UV-induced biochemical changes due to free radical proliferation in skin—DNA and cell membrane damage—associated with photo-aging and skin cancer. "These vitamins," points out Dr. Pathak, "may possibly act as UV absorbers as well. Important: PABA, a B vitamin that is the most widely used chemical sunscreen, is not effective as such in pill form."

Prevents Rashes, Blisters, Skin Eruptions

Beta-carotene, an orange-yellow pigment found in carrots and dark green vegetables, is an oral sunscreen of special interest to Dr. Pathak, "not only because it is a particularly powerful antioxidant but because it is generally regarded as safe even when taken in large doses over a long period."

Beta-carotene, which becomes concentrated in subcutaneous fat (the layer just beneath the skin) is used to treat people with extreme photosensitivity from a variety of causes. Dr. Pathak says the standard 90 milligrams daily of beta-carotene prescribed for photosensitive individuals helps to prevent rashes, blisters, and other skin eruptions that otherwise would occur after only a few minutes of sun exposure. "The only drawback to beta-carotene treatment for some people is that it gives skin a pale orange tinge, concentrated on the face and soles of the feet. Finally, anyone with a photosensitivity problem despite faithful use of an SPF 15 or higher sunscreen, should consult a physician."[9]

CATALYTIC CLEANSING—BABY SKIN AT ANY AGE

You can enjoy a skin that is forever young with the use of these catalytic cleansing programs as well as better care of the body envelope. When you uproot, loosen, dissolve, and wash away toxic debris, you regenerate your skin cells. When cleansed and nourished, they give more youthful support to your body covering. Result? You have a baby-smooth skin—at any age. You do deserve the best that Nature has to offer. Take it and de-age your skin and entire body.

─────────────── *HIGHLIGHTS* ───────────────

1. *To have a "forever young" skin, try catalytic cleansing of cellulite, the main cause of visible aging.*
2. *Just five simple steps, built into your daily routine, help free your body of cellulite.*
3. *Joyce N. was able to erase her wrinkles and become young again in just one weekend on a simple program.*
4. *Locate your skin problem and the proper catalytic cleansing remedy.*
5. *Use the simple methods recommended by a leading dermatologist to restore the bloom of youth to your skin . . . almost overnight.*

6. *Water is a major ingredient that will cleanse and rejuvenate your skin . . . if it is used properly as described.*

7. *Protect your skin from sun abuse, says a dermatology professor, and you will save it from destruction. He tells you how!*

8. *Sunscreens can save your skin, along with a set of twelve simple guidelines prepared by dermatologists.*

9. *Several vitamins, found in everyday foods, and available as supplements, may well act as sunscreens . . . from the inside out, says a highly respected dermatologist.*

Chapter 4

HOW TO BALANCE YOUR BLOOD PRESSURE WITH INTERNAL WASHING

High blood pressure (hypertension) is a reaction to the accumulation of wastes that are "bursting at the seams" to be eliminated. These toxins play havoc with your pressure, causing distressing and dangerous irregularities. To understand how wastes are to blame for this imbalance and how internal washing can restore normal levels, let's look closer at this internal situation.

WHAT DOES "BLOOD PRESSURE" MEAN?

Blood pressure refers to the amount of force exerted in the bloodstream as it passes through the arteries. When the left ventricle of your heart contracts, or squeezes down, it forces your blood out into the arteries. The major arteries then expand to receive the oncoming blood. In every individual, blood pressure normally goes up and down during the day and night, depending on a variety of factors, including activity level, diet, and emotions.

How Pressure Occurs

The muscular linings of your arteries resist the pressure; the blood is squeezed out into the smaller vessels of your body. Blood pressure is the combined amount of pressure the blood is under as a result of the pumping of the heart, the resistance of the arterial walls, and the closing of the heart valves.

How Is Blood Pressure Diagnosed?

There are two basic terms involved:

1. *Systolic Pressure.* The pressure at which your heart pumps blood through the arteries and put maximum pressure against their walls. It is the top figure in a diagnostic reading.

2. *Diastolic Pressure.* This is the minimum pressure, which occurs when your heart is at peak relaxation between beats and fills with blood; and pressure against the artery walls drops. This is the bottom figure in a diagnostic reading.

What Is a Normal Level?

A systolic/diastolic reading of "120 over 80" is considered to be normal.

What Are Risky Levels?

Doctors describe high blood pressure as mild, moderate, or severe. The diastolic (bottom) reading is usually used as the main indicator.

- *Borderline Hypertension* —A reading of 140/90
- *Mild Hypertension* —A reading of 170/105
- *Moderate Hypertension* —A reading of 185/115
- *Severe Hypertension* —A reading of 220/140 *and over*

BEWARE PROLONGED HYPERTENSION— THE SILENT KILLER

High blood pressure usually causes NO symptoms in the early stages. Only regular checkups can detect it. A majority of people with high blood pressure don't know they have it! This emphasizes the importance of regular physical checkups!

Everyone needs blood pressure. Each time your heart beats, it pumps blood through your arteries. The blood travels through the circulatory system to the organs and muscles of your body, carrying the oxygen and nutrients they need to perform their vital functions. The force of the blood being pushed through the arteries causes pressure against their walls. This pressure, which is generally measured in the artery of the upper arm, is your blood pressure.

Problem: When this pressure goes up and *stays up,* it causes hypertension. This places your heart and arteries under an abnormal amount of strain. The excess pressure constantly pounds all body organs nourished by the blood supply. Prolonged high blood pressure worsens any existing heart condition, forces the heart to work harder, and may also bring on the condition of atherosclerosis.

More Risks: A blood vessel in the brain may burst, causing a stroke. There is impairment of the kidneys' ability to filter out wastes, leading to toxic buildup. The heart, which must work harder to pump blood against the increased pressure in the arteries, may begin to show signs of strain. If ignored, high blood pressure can cause irreversible body injury.

Hypertensives have four times more heart attacks than those with normal blood pressure. And when a hypertensive does fall victim to such a heart attack, it is much more likely to be fatal. High blood pressure can also cause damage to the kidneys, eyes, and other organs. It can weaken the walls of the veins and arteries in the brain. This could result in a fatal or crippling stroke.

TOXIC WASTE OVERLOAD—BASIC CAUSE OF RUNAWAY BLOOD PRESSURE

The accumulation of toxic wastes is a key factor in erratic and runaway readings of blood pressure. Consuming synthetic foods, salt residue, artificial ingredients, excessive fats, and irritating stimulants (found in coffee, tea, soft drinks, and packaged beverages) all cause these toxic wastes to be deposited on the vital components of your cardiovascular system.

Toxins Cause Risky Rise in Pressure

Accumulation of these wastes creates deposits that stick stubbornly to the walls of your arteries. Glue-like, these toxins squeeze the channels through which blood and oxygen must travel to nourish your body. This situation still allows your heart and arteries to perform, but the choking action ultimately brings on the risk described by doctors as *congestive heart failure.* To protect against this threat to your health, your goal should be the internal washing of these sludge deposits clinging to your arteries. When cleansed, your arteries will function smoothly and you can then balance your blood pressure to enjoy a more energetic and youthful lifestyle.

Seven Steps to Scrub Away Sludge and Control Blood Pressure

You can control pressure with a set of seven steps, outlined by Edward D. Frohlich, M.D., vice-president for education and research, Alton Ochsner Medical Clinic of New Orleans, Louisiana.

1. *Avoid Overweight.* Reduce the pressure on your body caused by excess poundage. Too much weight increases tissue fluid volume and peripheral resistance. This leads to a rise in blood pressure. *Inner Cleansing Guidelines:* Try not to eat alone; this means faster eating and poor se-

lections. Plan meals as if you were eating with others. Listen to relaxing music to pass the time while you eat. Avoid high calorie foods such as those that are fried, very fatty, and heavily sweetened. Try to get family and friends to support your effort to lose weight. Let them know what your goal is and why it is important to your health.

2. *Avoid Smoking.* Nicotine, carcinogenic tars, and other pollutants enter your body through tobacco smoke—whether your own or sidestream. Your circulatory system becomes congested which causes severe pumping of blood and rise in pressure. *Inner Cleansing Guidelines:* Give up smoking. Not easy? Join a support group. Make a total commitment to kicking the habit. Keep away from others who smoke. You may have to go through several tries and failures before you finally succeed in quitting. This is a physical problem of addiction. With a structured strategy and group support, you can have victory over this body pollutant and trigger of spiralling pressure.

3. *Less Fatty Foods.* Dr. Edward Frohlich cautions that "fat may taste good, but excessive amounts of saturated fat is hurtful. Fat is a major villain in cardiovascular problems and that includes high blood pressure." *Inner Cleansing Guidelines:* Use just enough fat in cooking to induce flavor and make foods palatable. Cut out deep frying altogether. "This method of cooking can triple the calories in some foods. A better choice would be to stir-fry the food in a small amount of polyunsaturated vegetable oil." Beware hidden fats in snack foods (potato chips and processed goodies) as well as in many pastries and sweets.

4. *Moderate Alcohol Consumption.* Too much alcohol can raise your blood pressure. Alcoholic beverages often contain chemicals, artificial ingredients, colorings, and preservatives of which you are unaware since labels rarely give *all* ingredients and flavorings. You deposit unlimited sludge on your arteries with drinking. *Inner Cleansing Guidelines:* Dr. Frohlich says, "Because it is often hard to control high blood pressure in patients with high alcohol intake, we ask that you moderate your consumption. In order to avoid alcohol's effect on your blood pressure, I ask that you restrict yourself to no more than two ounces of ethanol per day. What that means in terms of popular alcoholic beverages is limiting yourself to four ounces of 100-proof whiskey, or 16 ounces of wine, or 48 ounces of beer." In a group, consider alternatives to alcoholic beverages such as fresh or sugar-free fruit juice, vegetable juice, herbal iced tea, sparkling spring water with a twist of fruit, or club soda with ice cubes and a lemon slice.

5. *Ease Arterial Pressure.* In some situations, the pressures from certain foods cause heart-thumping pressure on your arteries. Go easy on

whatever causes this increased pressure. *Inner Cleansing Guidelines:* Discuss any foods or situations that tend to upset your pressure with your health practitioner. With some adjustments, you can avoid this toxic assault upon your arteries and keep them clean and free-flowing.

6. *Reduce Sodium Intake.* "Are you salt sensitive?" asks Dr. Frohlich. "If so, your blood pressure may be high because of it." If your blood pressure is below 140/90, perhaps you can enjoy an occasional pretzel or two. But remember, you want to become immune to this condition so moderation is a key. Sodium is best reduced or eliminated for overall better health. *Inner Cleansing Guidelines:* Keep your salt shaker . . . but throw out the salt. Replace salt with flavorful herbs and spices. If you are eating out, order items lowest in sodium. The salad bar is generally a good choice, especially if you concentrate on the fresh fruits and vegetables. Avoid adding condiments such as canned chick peas and kidney beans, bacon bits, croutons, olives, and salted sunflower seeds. If you must use salt, about one-and-a-half teaspoons of salt each day is considered a safe amount. But, please, no more!

7. *Stress and Tension.* There is much evidence that lowering stress can help lower blood pressure, too. Stress causes internal pollution as a plethora of substances pour forth, depositing wastes on your vital organs. This causes erosion and subsequent deterioration of vital processes. For example, certain substances released during times of stress increase salt retention and slow down kidney excretion. They lower your body's resistance to sludge formation and diminish the efficacy of your detoxification mechanism. *Inner Cleansing Guidelines:* Steer clear of situations that make you stressful. Easier said than done, but with pre-planning, you can keep such clashes to a minimum. Keep yourself fit. Aerobic or oxygenating exercises that cause heavy breathing have a unique benefit: they stimulate the movement of the mucosal blanket that coats your respiratory tract and causes a filtering out of toxins. Intense exertion mobilizes fat in which toxic chemicals such as DDT and other pesticides are stored, making them available for excretion. Dr. Frohlich prescribes, "Regular, brisk, and sustained exercise such as brisk walking, jogging, and swimming improves the efficiency of your heart and burn off a lot of calories. You might also try jumping rope, stationary cycling, jogging, rowing. But remember, regular exercise means the activity is repeated at least three times per week."

Dr. Frohlich urges caution if there is a family history of premature cardiovascular fatalities, cardiac enlargement, protein-uria (protein in the urine), or serum creatinine (spillover of a protein metabolite into the bloodstream). Regular examinations are urged for any of these conditions whether in your family or yourself. With this seven-step inner cleansing program, you should be able to free yourself from circulation sludge and cleanse your arteries so that you can balance your blood pressure—and stay alive younger . . . and longer.[10]

NUTRITIONAL PROGRAMS TO TREAT HYPERTENSION

Sodium reduction is a standard practice for bringing down pressure readings. Follow through with a set of nutritional programs outlined by Stephen Brunton, M.D., director of family medicine, Long Beach (Calif.) Memorial Medical Center and clinical professor of Medicine, University of California at Irvine.

Minerals

"Controversy exists regarding the role of low levels of potassium, magnesium, and calcium in the development and maintenance of hypertension. Nevertheless, it would be prudent to maintain adequate levels of these important minerals."

Vegetarians, Fats in Diet

Dr. Brunton notes, "Vegetarians and persons with a diet high in polyunsaturated fats have been shown to have a lower blood pressure than those with a diet high in saturated fats and low in polyunsaturated fats."

Fish Oils Lower Pressure

Dr. Brunton also tells us, "It has been shown that ingesting 50 ml (three tablespoons) of fish oils per day for two months resulted in an average decline of 6.5 mm of systolic and 4.5 mm of diastolic blood pressure in hypertensives. These studies provide further impetus for recommending a heart-healthy diet."

Dr. Brunton concludes: "Using a non-pharmacologic approach to hypertension is an important adjunct for controlling blood pressure. Benefits may include not only reducing the need for medication, but also improving the subjective perception of well-being and increasing quality of life. It is important to monitor the progress of patients placed on a nondrug regimen."[11]

POTASSIUM—CLEANSING MINERAL

"The higher the potassium and the less of the sodium is one way to have a more balanced blood pressure," says Ray W. Gifford, Jr., M.D., director of regional health affairs with the Cleveland (Ohio) Clinic Foundation. "It may very well be beneficial as a non-pharmacological remedy. A potassium supplement may be very helpful."

Dr. Gifford says that along with potassium, follow the basic cleansing guidelines of low-salt, decreased alcohol, healthy weight, and regular monitoring of the condition.[12]

How Potassium Promotes Inner Cleansing and Lowers Pressure

This powerful mineral is an effective diuretic. It helps your body rid itself of excess water. It also helps slough off sodium, a beneficial effect called *natriuresis*. It appears to influence those physiological systems that regulate blood pressure and control the workings of the vascular system. There is reported evidence that the hypertensogenic (hypertension-causing) effect of excess sodium is counteracted by extra dietary potassium. Daily intake of potassium may well be a powerful form of inner cleansing to lower pressure. *Potassium Food Sources:* Cantaloupe, winter squash, potatoes, broccoli, orange juice, yogurt, brewer's yeast, wheat bran, parsnip, mushrooms, tomato, honeydew, apricots, bananas. *Careful:* potassium is water-soluble and can easily be lost in the cooking process. To minimize loss, steam rather than boil vegetables. For example, steamed vegetables lose only 3 percent to 6 percent, while boiled vegetables may lose up to 50 percent of their potassium. Wherever possible, eat raw fruits or vegetables (if they do not require cooking, obviously.)

GARLIC WASHES YOUR ARTERIES, BALANCES YOUR BLOOD PRESSURE

This miracle, lifesaving food has the power to uproot and dislodge the artery-choking sludge deposits and cast them out of your body. This opens the way for a balanced and lifesaving blood pressure.

Benjamin Lau, M.D., professor at California's Loma Linda University School of Medicine and a specialist in microbiology and immunology tells us that garlic can be part of your pressure-balancing program.

"Few drugs for controlling blood pressure are without side effects.

One of the most distressful side effects in the male patients is impotence. These patients become irritable, frustrated, and depressed." Dr. Lau tells how garlic has been used for centuries in Asia for treating hypertension. "One researcher tested 100 hypertensive patients by giving them initially large doses of garlic, gradually tapering the amount of garlic as the experiment progressed.

"After just one week of garlic treatment, forty of the patients had a drop of 20 mm Hg or more in their blood pressure. Other small-scale studies have shown similar positive effects of garlic on hypertension.

"In another study in China, 70 hypertensive patients were given the equivalent of 50 grams of raw garlic a day. Thirty-three of the patients showed a marked lowering of blood pressure; fourteen showed moderate reductions in blood pressure, for an overall success rate of 61.7 percent."

Dr. Lau tells of other situations in which garlic caused a systolic pressure drop of 20 to 30 mm Hg and a diastolic pressure drop of 10 to 20 mm Hg. "Patients also noted improvement of other physical symptoms, such as headaches, dizziness, angina-like chest pain and backaches." [13]

Cleans Arteries

When additional garlic is included in your daily food program, it is able to dissolve a harmful toxic waste that sticks to your low-density lipoprotein (LDL) factor. Garlic, because of its allicin content, scrubs away toxic wastes and cleanses arteries so you have better distribution of blood-carrying oxygen. By opening up arterial channels, there is a welcome relief from forced blood pumping, thus the pressure is restored to a healthier reading. Include garlic daily for this internal washing benefit.

Washes Clot Risk

In toxic overload, the glue-like wastes actually cause blood platelets to clump together. This platelet sludge can lead to a dangerous blood clot. Garlic comes to the rescue. It washes away the gluey sludge. Once the wastes are cleansed, the mobile platelets are liberated and do not loom as the risk of a clot. Again, by eating garlic daily, you can wash away this blood clot risk.

Improves Basic Circulation

A unique benefit of garlic is its power to increase a washing called *fibrinolyctic activity*. It exerts its allicin power along with its mitogenetic factor, which stimulates a healthy flow of blood. This allows your fibrins (protein-like substances) to become cleansed, free of sludge that otherwise would choke off circulation and predispose a risk of clotting. Clean fibrins = clean circulation = balanced blood pressure. You cause this inner cleansing with the circulation-washing garlic!

CIRCADIAN RHYTHMS MAY CAUSE MORNING DIZZINESS AND BLOOD PRESSURE RISE

Ticking away in every one of your cells is a biological clock which regulates every vital body process, says William Frishman, M.D., professor of medicine at New York's Albert Einstein College of Medicine. "Because of this rhythm, you are more prone to heart attacks in the morning."

Morning Pressure Is Highest

Dr. Frishman explains, "When you wake up, blood pressure, heart rate, contractibility goes up. It's a biological factor that allows you to get out of bed, to stand up. Your peripheral vessels have to work harder and pump more to allow you to start moving and to stand up. Blood is stickier in the morning. Catecholamines (neurotransmitters) go higher in the morning to prepare you for the day ahead. You are stimulated so that you can cope with the changes to come.

"On the other hand, blood pressure is lower when you are reclining. It is lower at night, hence the morning increase in platelet aggregation when you start moving. This may account for the dizziness you feel when you start to get out of bed. These daily cycles are known as circadian rhythms, from the term 'circa' (about) and 'dian' (day)."

See-Saw Pressure

Blood pressure appears to rise from a basal night-time level at or near the time of awakening. It remains at a day-time level until the night when it may come down appreciably. "There may be an association between the early morning rise in blood pressure and cerebral and coronary ischemic events (inadequate flow of blood to body part caused by constriction or blockage of the blood vessels supplying it). This rise in blood pressure may be caused by elevations in catecholamines and steroids from basal levels.[14]

Garlic at Night, Pressure Balance in Morning

To help ease this see-saw reaction, take a garlic clove at night. While you sleep, the released allicin tends to keep your pressure under reasonable balance. When you awaken, the time release of the allicin will make it easier for you to get out of bed and walk around with a minimum of dizziness or lightheadedness. Also . . . do NOT jump out of bed. Do it slowly. Start to walk very slowly so that your pressure evens out and you will feel more comfortable.

GARLIC + ONIONS = HEALTHY BLOOD PRESSURE

A combination of these two special vegetables can work cleansing miracles in providing you with a healthier blood pressure. *Unique Power:* Used in combination, both vegetables are able to (1) lower high levels of blood fats; and (2) reduce levels of fibrin, the substance that becomes clogged with wastes and may cause blood clotting.

Powerful Substance Is Super-Cell Cleanser

Onions contain a cell cleanser known as prostaglandin A_1. When you eat onions together with garlic, this super-cell cleanser is doubly invigorated (more than if onions are eaten alone) and works swiftly to create a fibrin-washing and lifesaving benefit.

Controls Dangerous Sludge

Garlic and onions (both members of the allium family) are able to control formation of a dangerous sludge known as *thromboxane.* This toxic waste causes platelet aggregation (clumping together). When this happens, pressure soars. A blood clot risk may be imminent. But eating garlic and onions daily will provide a buffering reaction to this threat. An even more vital benefit is that these miracle foods will wash away the thromboxane sludge and give you free-moving platelets—and a safe, sane, and healthy blood pressure level.

Plan to eat garlic daily, either chewed in clove form, or chopped fine and added to soups, stews, salads, casseroles, or baked foods. Combine garlic with onions in these recipes. You will be fortifying the metabolic system with the super-cleanser that protects against sludge buildup and gives you immunity from the risk of a fatal heart attack.

CASE HISTORY—"Dangerous" Pressure Drops Overnight

Kate H. was told by her cardiovascular specialist that she had a blood pressure reading of 200/150. This was so dangerous, she was given a 50-50 chance of survival! Medications made her dizzy and nauseous. She needed help swiftly. The doctor advised her to consume at least one whole head of garlic daily (either raw or cooked in any desired way) together with several onions for better assimilation. Kate H. followed this program. Overnight, the miracle combination actually "devoured" the sludge that was choking her arterioles and washed the wastes out of her body. Next day, Kate H. went in for another reading. The specialist told her happily that it had dropped to 150/95—almost normal. Kate H. felt she had been snatched from the jaws of hypertension-caused heart failure by the scrubbing action of garlic and onions.

THE LOW-SALT WAY TO WASTE-FREE ARTERIES AND NORMAL PRESSURE

Salt from the shaker or in processed foods is a major cause of toxic sludge. Certain substances in your blood become "coated" with salt residue. An excess of these cellular coatings can cause a stagnation that is the forerunner of high blood pressure.

Toxic Waste Reaction of Salt

When you consume salt, it encrusts your millions of cells. In this form, it builds up toxic wastes that narrow the passageways of your small arteries. This same waste will "choke" the glands to reduce hormone flow; this plays havoc with your blood pressure and basic health. Salt wastes also cause enlargement of the heart. This overload is more than a cause of hypertension; it is a cause of premature death!

Sneaky Reaction of Salt-Wastes

When salt-wastes increase, they block vital fluids in your circulatory system. This causes blood pressure to zoom to an unhealthy and dangerous high. CAUTION: Salt intake for a brief period of time (as minimal as one day) can trigger sludge overload and hypertension from the start. Avoid salt!

CASE HISTORY—"Restored to Life" on a "Glue-Free" Food Program

As a technician, Philip T. was under much business stress and strain, which undoubtedly contributed to his escalating blood pressure. His company physician said his excessive salt intake had caused "glue-like compounds" to "lock" the platelets together, choking off free blood circulation. Philip T. had a dangerously high reading of 260/150 that kept climbing. He was told if it went higher, it could be fatal! Swift action was needed to save his toxin-infested condition. He eliminated all forms of salt and sodium. He switched to flavorful herbs and spices. Within nine days, his pressure dropped to a healthful 130/80. In effect, he had been "restored to life" on this "glue-free" program that now keeps him alive and happy. Stress had something to do with his brush with death. Glue-forming salt was the villain!

SIX WAYS TO CLEAN YOUR ARTERIES AND BALANCE BLOOD PRESSURE

Sludge accumulation increases your risk of high blood pressure. But a few simple changes in your way of life (and eating) can help you wash out this sludge and keep it out so that you can clean your arteries and balance your pressure. The changes are easy to follow—lifesaving, too.

1. *Avoid Salt Sediment.* Keep this toxic "food" out of your home. Avoid its use in foods. Read labels of packaged foods and beware of their use. Use flavorful herbs and spices to give you the taste of sodium without its waste-clogging penalties.

2. *Boost Potassium Intake.* This mineral is an effective "blood washer." It boosts your catalytic response; that is, it activates "messages" through your nervous system to dispatch enzymes that dilute and wash wastes out of your system. Plan to eat high-potassium foods as outlined previously. Avoid sodium foods. You'll wash out blockages that threaten to raise blood pressure.

3. *Be Cautious About Hard Fats.* Animal (saturated) fats cling to your vital organs, choke off transportation of blood and oxygen. Use them moderately, if at all. Switch to polyunsaturated oils (in moderation, too; a little goes a long way.) They have valuable essential fatty acids that break up and wash away wastes.

4. *Unlock Blockage on a Caffeine-Free Program.* Coffee, tea, chocolate products, and many cola beverages and soft drinks contain heavy concentrations of caffeine. This drug-like substance distorts your nervous system, "chokes" your circulation, and deposits sediment at crucial points. It also boosts hypertension. Switch to coffee substitutes, herbal teas, carob confections (without sugar), and fresh juices. You will help unblock congestion and balance pressure.

5. *Less Weight = Less Blood Pressure.* Fat-encrusted cells and tissues cause excess weight: wash out burdensome fatty calories, control fat intake, limit caloric intake, exercise more. When you lose weight, you help your blood pressure work smoothly.

6. *Exercise Away Toxic Wastes.* Physical activities, simple exercises pep up your sluggish system. Fitness exercises will loosen stubborn toxic

wastes and prepare them for elimination. Shake clinging wastes "free" with exercise so they are washed out of your body. Your blood pumps more efficiently without these blockages. You are rewarded with healthful blood pressure and freedom from the threat of hypertension.

Build these simple six steps into your lifestyle. You will enjoy clean arteries and a balanced blood pressure.

THE "SNACK" THAT CONTROLS BLOOD PRESSURE

Obey the urge to snack—with garlic!

Carry a packet of garlic cloves in a small bottle. Whenever you want to snack, chew one clove thoroughly. You release a rich concentration of a trace mineral called *selenium*. This mineral combines with garlic's biologically active anti-atherosclerotic ingredients and works to prevent platelet adhesion or clot blockage. Selenium is then activiated by the garlic's ingredients to chip away and dissolve these adhesions or sediments and expel them from your body.

Unusual Benefit

When garlic is consumed without other foods, its volatile actions are super-concentrated. It works more vigorously without interference in washing away cellular debris. Garlic is better able to control blood pressure when taken alone. So you can indeed snack your way to a balanced blood pressure with powerful garlic.

CASE HISTORY—Saves His Life with Simple Daily Snack

"Either bring down that sky-high pressure, or get ready for a funeral . . . your own!" Those shocking words told Peter F. that his 300/220 reading could end his life at almost any moment. The problem was that this electrical engineer could not take medications. Side effects ranged from falling asleep at the wheel to painful spasms. He needed swift treatment. He discussed the problem with an orthomolecular (nutrition-minded) physician who outlined the preceding six step program—and told him to start snacking on garlic. He was to take at least four whole garlic cloves daily . . . one at a time, of course. Immediately, the frightened Peter F. started chewing on the garlic cloves. He boosted his intake to five whole garlic cloves daily "for good measure." In three days, his reading dropped to 180/120. In five days, he had a reading of 125/80. His blockage had been dislodged and eliminated by the garlic ingredients. This miracle vegetable had saved his life, all with simple daily snacks.

WASH AWAY HYPERTENSION . . . WITHOUT DELAY

Don't let it fool you. Hypertension is an ailment without symptoms, a "silent executioner." If you don't control it, then it could lead to a heart attack, stroke, or kidney failure. You must nip hypertension in the bud. Get to the root of the problem—toxic waste accumulations that prematurely age the body and strike down its victims. Internal washing is the key to overcoming this dangerous threat.

High blood pressure is compared to a "time bomb" ticking away in your body. Don't wait until it goes off. Wash away that debris right now . . . while you still have time.

—————— *HIGHLIGHTS* ——————

1. *Familiarize yourself with blood pressure and learn how internal cleansing can save your life.*

2. *Scrub away pressure-causing sludge with the set of seven steps outlined by a leading physician.*

3. *Nutritional remedies help control pressure readings.*

4. *Potassium is a powerful cleansing mineral that lowers pressure. It is easily available in many foods.*

5. *Garlic washes your arteries, balances your pressure. Combine with onions as a double miracle in cleansing and pressure control.*

6. *Overcome morning reactions with garlic the night before.*

7. *Kate H. saw her dangerous pressure drop overnight.*

8. *Avoid salt—it deposits sludge in your bloodstream and raises pressure. Follow salt-quitting suggestions.*

9. *Avoid "glue-forming" products. Philip I. was "restored to life" on this simple program.*

10. *Wash away toxins and balance pressure on a simple six-step program.*

11. *Garlic as a snack saved Peter F. from threatening fatality.*

Chapter 5

HOW TO PUT NEW YOUTH INTO YOUR TIRED DIGESTIVE SYSTEM

A sparkling clean set of digestive organs is your key to total youth. Digestion is the process by which your body dissolves food, breaking it down into simpler substances which are absorbed by your blood and used for energy.

Normally, the organs and glands of the digestive tract work like an efficient assembly line. When you eat, food you swallow drops down the esophagus into your stomach, where it is mixed with gastric juices containing acid and enzymes. In less than an hour, your stomach begins pushing the food through the pyloric sphincter into the duodenum, where it is bathed in digestive juices secreted by the liver and the pancreas.

From there, the partially digested food travels through the small intestine, where more enzymes break down proteins, fats, and starches into food molecules which are absorbed into the bloodstream. Undigested food and waste products move into the large intestine, or colon.

Internal Toxemia Causes Problems

Healthy organs transform foods into nutrients that nourish and regenerate your body from head to toe. If these organs become clogged with wastes, their efficiency is decreased. They cannot completely metabolize foods; they become weak in their task of assimilating youth-building elements. This leads to general body decline and loss of vital responses. If the digestive organs become excessively saturated with glue-like wastes, premature aging begins. Health slips away, bit by bit.

To protect yourself against this undesirable risk, you need to cleanse away toxic wastes from your organs and allow them to perform smoothly and efficiently in helping you enjoy healthy digestion and total youth.

HOW TO WASH AWAY THE "GLUE" THAT CAUSES CONSTIPATION

An accumulation of "glue-like" wastes from improperly digested refined foods is often the cause of the blockage known as constipation. Your intestinal membranes become choked with artificial deposits from refined products as well as the sludge of sugar and salt. These toxins clump together to create wedges that block the release of wastes. How do you get them out? In a word—*fiber.*

How Fiber Is Good for Your Digestive System

Fiber is necessary to maintain normal functioning of the gastrointestinal tract. It helps to correct constipation and other disorders. High-fiber meals provide a feeling of satiety which can help dieters keep their portions small. A high-fiber diet protects against colon cancer by diluting potential carcinogens and removing them quickly from the body. For diabetics, a high-fiber diet, rich in complex carbohydrates, improves control of blood sugar and may reduce the amount of medication needed.

What Is Fiber?

Fiber is not a single substance. Rather, it is a complex mixture of plant food materials that are resistant to digestion and pass through the intestines without being absorbed. For inner cleansing of wastes, focus on *insoluble* fiber, which is derived from the structural components of plant cell walls.

How Insoluble Fiber Washes Away "Glue"

When you ingest insoluble fiber, it absorbs water as it moves through your intestines, thus increasing the bulk of stools, reducing the "transit time" of glue materials through your system. This helps create a form of inner cleansing that washes away the glue to prevent an array of gastrointestinal-related disorders such as spastic colon, diverticulitis, and hemorrhoids. Basic insoluble fiber sources include fruit and vegetable skins, whole-grain products such as bran (especially wheat bran), and some seeds.

How Much Fiber Daily?

The ideal fiber intake has not been established. A conservative estimate of the insoluble fiber intake required to promote the health of the gastrointestinal tract would be 15 grams per day. You might aim for about 25 or 30 grams to help boost inner cleansing. *Careful:* Don't overdo it—too much fiber may cause colon obstruction, although such situations are infrequent. Be sure to drink lots of water when taking fiber foods as part of a balanced food program. See the checklist of fiber foods and plan your daily menu around this wide and tasty variety.

FIBER CONTENT OF FOOD
(IN GRAMS)

FRUITS

	Serving Size	Fiber (g.)		Serving Size	Fiber (g.)
Apple (w/skin)	1 med.	3.5	Mango	1 med.	3.0
Apricot	1 med.	0.5	Nectarine	1 med.	1.0
Avocado	½ med.	3.0	Orange	1 med.	2.6
Banana	1 med.	2.4	Papaya	½ med.	1.5
Blackberries	½ cup	5.0	Peach (w/skin)	1	1.9
Blueberries	½ cup	2.0	Pear (w/skin)	½ large	3.1
Cantaloupe	¼ melon	1.0	Pineapple	½ cup	1.0
Cherries, sweet	10	1.2	Plum	1 small	0.5
Cranberries	½ cup	1.0	Prunes	3	3.0
Dates	5 med.	2.0	Raisins	¼ cup	3.1
Figs	1 med.	1.7	Raspberries	½ cup	3.1
Grapefruit	½ med.	1.0	Rhubarb	½ cup	0.5
Grapes	½ cup	1.0	Strawberries	1 cup	3.0
Honeydew	½ small	2.0	Watermelon	1 cup	1.0

VEGETABLES

	Serving Size	Fiber (g.)		Serving Size	Fiber (g.)
Artichoke	1 med.	4.0	Onions	½ cup	1.0
Asparagus, cut	½ cup	1.0	Parsnips	½ cup	2.7
Beets	½ cup	0.5	Peas	½ cup	2.0
Broccoli	½ cup	2.2	Potato (w/skin)	1 med.	2.5
Brussels Sprouts	½ cup	2.3	Pumpkin	½ cup	1.5
Cabbage, common	1 cup	1.0	Spinach	1 cup	1.2
Cabbage, red	1 cup	2.0	Squash (summer)	½ cup	1.0
Carrot	1 med.	1.5	Squash (winter)	½ cup	2.0
Cauliflower	½ cup	1.0	String Beans, green	½ cup	1.6
Celery, diced	½ cup	1.1	Sweet Potato	½ med.	1.5
Cucumber	½ cup	0.4	Tomato	1 med.	1.5
Eggplant	½ cup	0.5	Turnip	½ cup	1.6
Lettuce, sliced	1 cup	0.9	Yam	½ cup	1.0
Mushrooms	½ cup	1.5	Zucchini	½ cup	1.8

LEGUMES

	Serving Size*	Fiber (g.)		Serving Size	Fiber (g.)
Baked beans	½ cup	8.8	Lima beans	½ cup	4.5
Black-eyed peas	½ cup	2.5	Navy beans	½ cup	6.0
Dried peas	½ cup	4.7	Pinto beans	½ cup	2.5
Green beans	½ cup	1.6	Split peas	½ cup	2.5
Kidney beans	½ cup	7.3	White beans	½ cup	2.5
Lentils	½ cup	3.7	*(All servings ½ cup after cooking.)		

BREADS AND PASTAS

	Serving Size	Fiber (g.)		Serving Size	Fiber (g.)
Bagel	1	0.6	Italian bread	1 slice	0.5
Bagel (whole wheat)	1	1.2	Macaroni	1 cup	0.5
Biscuit	1	0.5	Oatmeal bread	1 slice	0.5
Bran muffin	1	2.5	Pumpernickel bread	1 slice	1.4
Bread stick	1	0.2	Spaghetti, cooked	½ cup	1.1
French bread	1 slice	0.7	Whole wheat bread	1 slice	2.0

NUTS AND SEEDS

	Serving Size	Fiber (g.)		Serving Size	Fiber (g.)
Almonds	10 nuts	1.1	Peanut butter	1 tbsp.	0.3
Cashews	1 cup	2.0	Pecans	1 cup	2.0
Chestnuts	1 cup	1.9	Pistachios	1 cup	2.0
Filberts	10 nuts	0.8	Pumpkin seeds	1 cup	2.0
Macadamia nuts	1 cup	2.0	Sunflower seeds	1 cup	2.0
Peanuts	10 nuts	1.4	Walnuts	1 cup	2.0

COLD CEREALS

	Serving Size	Fiber (g.)		Serving Size	Fiber (g.)
All-Bran	1 oz.	8.5	Honeycomb	1 oz.	0.4
Alpha-Bits	1 oz.	1.0	Life	1 oz.	0.9
Bran Buds	1 oz.	7.9	100% Bran	1 oz.	8.4
Bran Chex	1 oz.	6.1	Puffed Rice	1 oz.	0.0
Cap'n Crunch	1 oz.	0.3	Puffed Wheat	1 oz.	0.0
Cheerios	1 oz.	2.0	Raisin Bran	1 oz.	3.0
Cocoa Puffs	1 oz.	0.0	Rice Chex	1 oz.	0.3
Corn Bran	1 oz.	5.4	Rice Krispies	1 oz.	1.0
Corn Flakes	1 oz.	0.3	Shredded Wheat	1 oz.	3.2
Cracklin' Bran	1 oz.	4.3	Special K	1 oz.	0.0
Frosted Flakes	1 oz.	0.6	Total	1 oz.	2.0
Fruit & Fibre	1 oz.	3.0	Trix	1 oz.	0.1
Golden Grahams	1 oz.	0.5	Wheat Chex	1 oz.	2.1
Grape-nuts	1 oz.	1.8	Wheaties	1 oz.	2.0

MISCELLANEOUS

	Serving Size	Fiber (g.)		Serving Size	Fiber (g.)
Apple juice	1 cup	1.0	Orange juice	1 cup	1.0
Blueberry muffin	1 avg.	0.5	Pancake	1 avg.	0.5
Bran muffin	1 avg.	2.5	Popcorn, popped	1 cup	1.0
Brown rice, cooked	1 cup	2.0	Potato chips	2 oz.	1.0
Corn chips	2 oz.	1.0	Saltines	2	0.2
Grape juice	1 oz.	0.0	White rice, cooked	1 cup	1.0

OTHER FOODS

Dairy products, fats and oils, and **meats and fish** contain no dietary fiber. **Poultry** has small amounts (under 1 gram per serving).

Herbs and spices do contain fiber, but because we ingest them in minuscule quantities, it is difficult to pick up measurable amounts of fiber from them.

Beer, alone among alcoholic beverages, contains fiber: about 1 gram per 12 oz. serving.

The fiber content of **soup** varies according to its ingredients. Soups thick with beans or potatoes can contain as much as 3 grams of fiber per bowl. Most others contain 1 gram or less.

Most **hot cereals** contain negligible amounts of dietary fiber. Exceptions include oatmeal (about 1.5 grams per serving) and Ralston Purina (about 3.5 grams per serving).

POTASSIUM: THE MINERAL THAT OPENS UP TIGHT INTESTINAL ORGANS

Potassium is a waste-washing and organ-scrubbing mineral that opens up clogged intestinal organs. It initiates a gentle but effective contraction of the toxic-burdened sphincter muscles, helping to dislodge accumulated wastes.

Potassium further penetrates the intestinal cells and tissues of these muscles, revitalizing them to perform their organ-scrubbing responsibilities. Within moments, the stored-up contents are being readied for removal.

Sources of organ-scrubbing potassium are green leafy vegetables, oranges, whole grains, potatoes (especially the skin), bananas, apple cider vinegar, sun-dried apricots, figs, and prunes.

THE 25-CENT FRUIT THAT CREATES SWIFT WASTE-WASHING

The humble-looking prune is a powerhouse of potassium to detoxify your inner organs. Just a few prunes in the morning, at a cost of a quarter or less, can boost this organ-scrubbing action to overcome constipation. Add some pitted prunes with fresh fruits to a bowl of whole-grain cereal with skim milk or fruit juice . . . and you detoxify in a matter of moments.

X
How to Clean Your Digestive System in Moments

In the morning, pour two cups of freshly boiled water over a few sun-dried prunes. In minutes, they will "plump" up, making it easier to remove the pits. When lukewarm, eat the prunes and then slowly sip the liquid. Do this on an empty stomach before breakfast.

Melts Glue, Unlocks Sludge, Removes Wastes The high concentration of potassium works with vitamin A (abundant in prunes in the form of beta-carotene) to stimulate the enzymatic process. This melts down the glue-like wastes, dissolves the blockages, and propels them to eliminative channels. The lukewarm juice is a powerhouse of potassium and enzymes that further work to scrub your intestines and free them of the toxic wastes that have become "pasted" together to cause constipation.

FIGS HELP BOOST INNER CLEANSING VIA AMAZING FIBER CONTENT

California fresh figs, available in many fresh produce outlets and health stores are rich concentrates of a unique type of fiber. The figs have the fiber within their tiny seeds. When you eat several California fresh figs and drink a fresh fruit juice or other favorite natural beverage, the seeds become lique-fied and the fiber expands very gently so that the scrubbing action works with comfort and efficiency.

Several figs "the night before" or early in the morning will boost inner cleansing so that the wastes are actually scrubbed out of your body to improve the efficiency of your digestive system

CASE HISTORY—**Corrects Lifelong Constipation in Three Days**

Years of toxic waste overload made Dorothy P. feel miserable with her stubborn constipation. As a schoolteacher, she was sluggish in the morning when she had to be especially alert to teach her class. Laxatives weakened her intestines, not to mention causing embarrassment at the most inconvenient times. She was constantly "clogged up," had "sour stomach," and gas-like stomach rumbles. Dorothy P. was so clogged, she developed sallow, sagging skin and a frown. A sympathetic teacher suggested she consult a gastroenterologist. This doctor advised her to try the morning prune program . . . and alternate with figs in the same manner. Results: In only three days, the prune-fig remedy unblocked her toxic overload. She was free from lifelong constipation . . . and for only about 25 cents each morning. She felt reborn! Her skin cleared up and she was smiling happily. Dorothy P. discovered that "clean insides" will help create "youthful outsides."

HERBAL TREATMENTS TO CORRECT IRREGULARITY

Fiber and regular exercise are important for inner cleansing and healthily functioning bowels. Tension and emotional worries are negative responses so avoid these threats to your digestive health. You can use herbs to relieve irregularity. For example:

- One-half teaspoon of crushed flaxseed in a cup of freshly boiled water has a cleansing action which brings relief. Drink one cup in the morning and another in the evening. Add a twist of lemon or lime for a tangy taste.
- Licorice root (from a herbalist and *not* the chemicalized candy) is a mild and pleasant cleanser. Chew the root as desired. Or, make a decoction of 1 teaspoon root in a cup of boiled water and sip three times a day.
- Rose hips tea is also a mild cleanser. Strain the rose hips through filter paper to remove the seeds and tiny hairs which may be irritating. Drink whenever necessary.

HERBS THAT CLEANSE YOUR SYSTEM AND SOOTHE DIGESTION

Most flavoring and seasoning herbs and spices promote the flow of digestive enzymes in the stomach and intestine. This increases the efficiency with which fats are broken down into fatty acids and nutrients are absorbed by your body. For example, rosemary helps digest fatty lamb; fennel assists the digestion of oily fish; horseradish aids in digestion of beef. Try using the following herbs and spices to soothe your digestive system:

- One tablespoon ground aniseed added to one cup of milk. Drink twice a day to revive your digestive system.
- Comfortably hot peppermint tea taken after a meal will boost cleansing and a feeling of relaxation.

- Cardamom increases the flow of salivary enzymes and also adds a pleasant aroma that improves digestion. Take one cup of cardamom tea half an hour before each meal.
- End a heavier meal with spices and herbs such as aniseed, caraway, dill, and fennel seed.

SIX WAYS TO OVERCOME CONSTIPATION . . . NATURALLY!

Marvin Schuster, M.D., chief of the division of digestive diseases with the Baltimore (Maryland) City Hospitals, tells us, "Doctors agree that prevention is the best approach to constipation. While there is no way to ensure that you will never experience constipation, the following six guidelines should help:

1. Know what is normal for you and do not rely on laxatives unnecessarily.
2. Eat a well-balanced diet that includes unprocessed bran, whole wheat, prunes and figs, as well as their juices.
3. Drink plenty of fluids.
4. Exercise regularly.
5. Set aside time after breakfast or dinner to allow for undisturbed visits to the bathroom.
6. Never ignore the urge.

"Above all, it is necessary to recognize that a successful treatment program requires persistent effort and time."[15]

Bran to the Cleansing Rescue

Some doctors recommend adding *small* amounts of unprocessed bran to baked goods, cereals, and fruits as a way of increasing the fiber content of your diet. (Also known as "miller's bran," unprocessed bran is usually sold in health food stores or in the health foods section of supermarkets. It should not be confused with the packaged cereals that contain large amounts of bran or bran flakes.) You may have some bloating and gas for several weeks after adding bran to your program. But aside from this, it has a comfortable cleansing action. Remember, all changes should be made slowly, to allow your digestive system to adapt. *Important:* be sure to drink plenty of liquids . . . at least two quarts daily, to ease the bran reaction.

THE "MIRACLE SALAD" THAT REJUVENATES YOUR DIGESTIVE SYSTEM

The grime that clings stubbornly to your digestive-eliminative organs is comparable to thick grease on a pipe. It grows in bulk until it chokes off flow through the pipe. So it is with your digestive organs. An overload of accumulation of toxic wastes will so clog your vital organs that your entire digestive-assimilative functions become weakened. This leads to health-draining nutritional deficiencies that make you susceptible to the aging process. This need not happen. With the use of a special "miracle salad" you can rid yourself of intestinal stagnation and invigorate your vital organs with a "full steam ahead" scrubbing pace. You are then able to enjoy total youth with total nutrition.

"Miracle Salad"—How It Promotes Swift Cleansing

Combine a few chopped garlic cloves with an assortment of green leafy vegetables Add a few slices of raw onion. Sprinkle with two or three tablespoons of apple cider vinegar and a bit of oil. Mix together. Eat this "miracle salad" *before* your main meal. If you wish, add some slices of natural cheese with some bran or wheat germ Together with whole grain bread, it becomes a meal in itself.

Cleansing Benefits

The allicin in garlic is invigorated by the minerals in the onion. In this combination, the allicin penetrates the large intestine, bringing along the roughage of the raw green vegetables. The high potassium content of the apple cider vinegar boosts enzymatic action of the allicin. This dynamic garlic nutrient stimulates the peristaltic movement of your sluggish waste-covered intestinal walls. Almost at once, the allicin is able to dislodge the accumulated wastes and bring about swift cleansing.

A Salad a Day Keeps You Youthfully Clean Forever

This simply prepared "miracle salad" keeps you clean forever if eaten daily. The dynamic garlic allicin compound actually dissolves accumulated toxic wastes and helps to speedily eliminate them. You respond with more vigorous digestive action and improved assimilation of vital youth-building nutrients.

CASE HISTORY—**How "Miracle Salad" Promoted "Total Youth" in Four Days**

Internal sludge caused such intestinal blockage that Norah V. had a sallow look, complained of fatigue by the early afternoon, was unable to relax, and developed a skin outbreak. Her dermatologist diagnosed the problem as intestinal blockage. The toxic wastes were releasing putrid fumes that caused cellular deterioration as well as collagen disintegration. She needed speedy elimination of toxic wastes. The doctor prescribed the "miracle salad" to be eaten after her noon meal and then again after her dinner. Norah V. followed the program hopefully . . . desperately. The first day, she experienced long-awaited relief. The next day, she had more energy. Her blemishes were subsiding. The third day, her complexion became youthfully smooth. She felt energetic. At night, she enjoyed refreshing sleep. By the fourth day, she was so invigorated, she felt like a youngster again. The "miracle salad" had restored regularity and regenerated her powers of assimilation. Now she enjoyed "total youth," and it happened in four days.

Unplug Constipation with More Roughage

The sweeping action of enzyme-rich raw vegetables together with whole grains (containing wheat germ and bran) will unplug blockages and relieve constipation. Roughage/fiber helps to scrub your digestive system and to give you the refreshing look and feel of youth . . . at any age.

HOW TO WASH AWAY THE IRRITANTS OF INDIGESTION

Indigestion refers to symptoms that can be traced to toxic irritation caused by gastrointestinal blockage. You know you have indigestion when you feel "heartburn" (burning pain in your chest). Symptoms may include nausea, regurgitation, abdominal fullness or bloating after a meal, and stomach discomfort or pain. It suggests that you need to wash away the irritants to enjoy a sparkling clean digestive system.

Six Ways to End Problems of Indigestion

The moment toxic substances penetrate your system, your body reacts by trying to neutralize and/or excrete them. Your body is a natural detoxification center. How effectively this center works to neutralize, transform, and wash out toxins depends on better self-care. A few adjustments in your eating methods can control the accumulation of toxic wastes that cause indigestion. These include—

1. *Do not overeat.* Excessive indulgence will overwork your digestive enzymes so that they cannot break down food quickly. Decomposition of food occurs, which gives rise to toxic wastes and corrosive fumes. Eat moderately.

2. *Do not eat or drink too fast.* Gulped-down food that is improperly enzyme-digested will "rot" and bring on digestive upset. Eat at a leisurely pace; drink slowly. Your digestive system is better able to accommodate these foods and will not protest.

3. *Do not swallow excessive air.* Called *aerophagia,* the gulping of air through the mouth while taking in food will upset the internal oxygenation of your system. This disturbs the enzymatic balance and causes poor digestion, which leads to decomposed foods—the source of indigestion. Eat slowly and comfortably to reduce air intake.

4. *Chew your food thoroughly.* Thorough chewing ensures that the enzymes in saliva prepare swallowed food for more thorough digestion. Your digestive enzymes will be able to work more effectively on thoroughly chewed food. This avoids backup of chunks of decomposed and toxin-causing foods.

5. *Cook as thoroughly as required.* Undercooked food is difficult to digest; it causes indigestion through deposition of tough fibrous wastes that cling to your organs. Make it a rule to cook certain foods thoroughly. If the food must be cooked, do so!!

6. *Limit fat intake.* Animal fat is a major source of toxic waste accumulation. Greasy, it clings in clumps or droplets to vital digestive (and body) organs. Since grease and water do not mix, these wastes remain resistant and they accumulate stubbornly. To minimize this threat, limit your intake of animal fats. Trim away fat from meats before and after cooking. *Rule:* complete a meal with a fresh raw fruit platter for dessert. Excellent choices are papayas and pineapples, along with other fruits. The raw fruit enzymes are powerful, able to wash away grease and keep your digestive apparatus in a clean condition.

With these detoxification guidelines, you should be able to protect yourself against distressing indigestion.

HOW TO WASH AWAY THE PAIN OF ULCERS

An ulcer is a hole or an erosion in the tissue lining almost anywhere in the digestive tract. Ulcers are found most frequently in the duodenum and stomach. This crater-like sore in the thin membrane lining is caused by the corrosive effect of accumulated wastes that stubbornly refuse to be washed away. Often, these wastes release acid, which further erodes the digestive tract lining and erupts in ulcer formation. That is, an ulcer occurs when the lining is unable to resist the damaging effects of the acid and pepsin (an enzyme) produced by the stomach to digest foods.

Ulcers Are Destructive

Don't think that ulcers are harmless. Untreated ulcers can, and do, kill thousands of people every year through serious complications such as bleeding and peritonitis, an infection of the abdominal lining which can occur when an ulcer perforates the stomach wall.

Ulcers are caused by corrosive hydrochloric acid—this stomach acid is actually capable of eating through shoe leather!

It is believed that ulcers occur when there is an imbalance between the acid and pepsin found in the stomach and the normal defense factors that prevent the acid and pepsin from eating away the stomach lining!

To wash away the pain of ulcers, your goal is to wash away the acid-releasing waste accumulations. This sludge causes "internal spontaneous combustion," which gives off noxious vapors that cause this burning of the thin membrane lining the vital digestive organs. Detoxify the sludge and you help resolve the painful problem of ulcers.

Cabbage Juice—Cools Acid, Promotes Healing

An enzymatic ingredient found in freshly made cabbage juice functions as a natural antacid; a cooling-healing reaction is felt within a day or so. You must use *fresh* cabbage. If wilted or spoiled cabbage is used, the effect is weaker. You can juice cabbage with an electric extractor and have a glass or two in a jiffy. Be sure to drink the cabbage juice immediately after its preparation. Even if refrigerated for a day or two, the juice loses some of its potency. *Cooked* cabbage, although healthful, seems to lose the factor that detoxifies debris, cools the acid, and promotes healing.

CASE HISTORY—Magic Drink Ends Ulcer Distress

Gnawing ulcer pain turned Morton G. into a social and business loser. He rarely participated in local activities because the agonizing, burning pain in his stomach made him want to curl up in the seclusion of his bedroom. He became so wracked with pain that he could not devote full attention to his sales work as a route manager. Understandably, his career suffered as much as his health! Morton G. went the route of various medications which eased the pain, but once the drug wore off, the burning agony returned with vengeful intensity. At times, he lamented that he was being "burned alive" by the horrifying pain. A company internist suggested he follow a detoxification program that had helped banish ulcer agony for many others. Morton G. was to go on a program that would omit irritants. Whatever irritated him was to be omitted—including any seasonings, coffee, tea, whatever. Morton G. was also told to drink up to four glasses of freshly prepared cabbage juice made with an extractor.

He began the program a skeptic. Immediately, the juice gave him a soothing, balm-like contentment. Within four days, he could say goodbye and good riddance to the plague of ulcer pain. He began to enjoy a social and business life. He felt rejuvenated because of the detoxifying/healing power of the cabbage juice. When asked about his secret, he patted his now-soothed stomach smilingly and said it was a "magic drink." It had, indeed, brought on a magic healing.

Chew Your Way to Ulcer Detoxification

Thorough chewing is a unique way of detoxifying the hurtful sludge so that ulcer healing follows. Chewing releases an enzyme-like cleanser via your salivary glands called *urogastrone*. This enzyme cleanser has the ability to detoxify and scrub away wastes, then offer a protective balm coating your intestinal lining to protect against membrane erosion. Chewing protects against volatile gastric acidity, which irritates the sore on the membrane. Therefore, you can clean away the sludge and simultaneously initiate healing with the use of the urogastrone method. How? Simply chew all food thoroughly before swallowing. You'll soon be rewarded with a detoxified digestive system and a contented-cooled-cured ulcer.

Easy On Stress

There is controversy over whether stress actually causes ulcers. But if you already have an ulcer, stress worsens the condition. Stress is a cause of toxic overload. It is not so much the stressful event, but your reaction to it. To minimize stress, think pleasant thoughts. Frequently take five or more deep breaths to immediately oxygenate your system and induce calming. Regular exercise is a good coping mechanism. Relax your body and you relax your mind—and vice versa. It helps detoxify your system and ease ulcer unrest.

Avoid Whatever Burns You

Any disturbance of the delicate balance between the aggressive forces of the digestive process and the defensive forces of the stomach will lead to toxic overload and ulcer distress. *Beware:* Smoking, aspirin, and many nonsteroidal anti-inflammatory drugs (used to treat arthritis but may also damage the stomach lining) can cause erosions and ulcers. Sodium bicarbonate (in antacids) delivers an overload of sodium. Chronic alcohol consumption can irritate digestive tract membranes. These substances deposit toxic wastes which are the forerunner of ulcers. Basically, if it bothers you, keep away from it!!

Rearrange Meal Frequency

For many, three average size meals are fine, but others may have less ulcer distress if they consume smaller meals. Food helps neutralize stomach acid so six small meals daily may help in the detoxification program. Always begin your meal with a raw vegetable salad. End with a raw fruit platter. This will enable catalytic washing of your wastes to cleanse and heal your ulcerous wounds.

Clean your digestive system, and be rewarded with a sparkling metabolism that will give you the glow of the joy of youthful health.

HIGHLIGHTS

1. *"Gluelike" accumulations in your digestive organs contribute to toxic constipation. Use remedies listed to wash out the glue and enjoy inner cleanliness.*
2. *Use a simple 25-cent fruit to open up tight intestinal organs and promote speedy regularity.*
3. *See the fiber chart and read how to use this guide to detoxify and clean your insides.*
4. *Potassium is a "magic mineral" that opens up tight intestinal organs.*
5. *Herbal remedies detoxify the system and correct irregularity.*
6. *Dorothy P. conquered years of toxic waste overload constipation in just three days with a simple fruit program.*
7. *Overcome constipation naturally with the doctor-recommended set of six easy guidelines.*
8. *A "miracle salad" rejuvenates your digestive system speedily.*
9. *Scrub away digestive grime with the easy remedy used by Norah V. It gave her the look of "total youth" within four days.*
10. *Detoxify waste-irritating sludge that causes indigestion with an easy-to-follow six-step plan.*

11. *Wash away the pain of ulcers with a simple vegetable juice. Morton G. called it his "magic drink" because it ended his painful distress.*

12. *Chew your way to ulcer detoxification. As for eating guidelines: whatever burns you, avoid it!*

Chapter 6

FOODS AND JUICES THAT FLUSH AWAY OVERWEIGHT

Wash the fatty wastes out of your cells and become slim forever. These accumulations are the root cause of your stubbornly clinging excess weight. With the use of everyday foods and juices, you can break down weight-causing toxic wastes and flush the obesity right out of your body.

Certain foods release a catalytic enzyme reaction that melts and washes away the cellular wastes. This reaction is set off when fresh raw fruits and vegetables metabolize and release fat-melting enzymes that scrub and scour your cells, slimming them down. In effect, you can use foods to wash away overweight. Let's see how you can make this happen.

CELLULAR OVERLOAD—REAL CAUSE OF OVERWEIGHT

Overweight occurs when you have an excess of fatty wastes stored in your adipose (fat) cells and your adipose tissue. These adipocytes (fatty cells and tissues) are different from ordinary cells. Most of your normal cells contain a large amount of cytoplasm (gelatin-like substance), with the nucleus near the center of the cell.

Fat Cells Are Different

The composition of adipocytes is different. Fatty wastes make up almost the entire area of the cell. Once this penetration is allowed to accumulate, the cytoplasm and nucleus are displaced. That is, the stored-up sediment and sludge actually push out the movable cytoplasm and glue themselves to the adipocytes. More and more sludge fetters onto the already sticky sediment, and weight accumulates.

Obesity Continues to Expand

A swelling and proliferation of adipocytes occurs; this increases the amount of adipose tissue, ultimately erupting in ever-expanding obesity. To control this obesity and to help turn the tide, you need to scrub away these wastes from your adipocytes. You need to slim down your cells. Your body will correspondingly slim down, too. This is the root cause of your obesity. Your plan is to correct this cause, empty and scrub the fat-filled cells, and head toward lifetime slimness.

Before you begin, check your weight against the chart below. Set your goal. Make your plans. Become determined to cleanse your cells for a slimmer and healthier figure.

STANDARD HEIGHT AND WEIGHT CHART

MEN

Height (without shoes)	Weight (without clothing)		
	Light Build	Medium Build	Heavy Build
5 ft. 3 in.	118	129	141
5 ft. 4 in.	122	133	145
5 ft. 5 in.	126	137	149
5 ft. 6 in.	130	142	155
5 ft. 7 in.	134	147	161
5 ft. 8 in.	139	151	166
5 ft. 9 in.	143	155	170
5 ft. 10 in.	147	159	174
5 ft. 11 in.	150	163	178
6 ft.	154	167	183
6 ft. 1 in.	158	171	188
6 ft. 2 in.	162	175	192
6 ft. 3 in.	165	178	195

WOMEN

Height (without shoes)	Light Build	Medium Build	Heavy Build
5 ft.	100	109	118
5 ft. 1 in.	104	112	121
5 ft. 2 in.	107	115	125
5 ft. 3 in.	110	118	128
5 ft. 4 in.	113	122	132
5 ft. 5 in.	116	125	135
5 ft. 6 in.	120	129	139
5 ft. 7 in.	123	132	142
5 ft. 8 in.	126	136	146
5 ft. 9 in.	130	140	151
5 ft. 10 in.	133	144	156
5 ft. 11 in.	137	148	161
6 ft.	141	152	166

FOOD ENZYMES WASH AWAY FATTY WASTES

Fresh raw fruits and vegetables and their fresh juices are powerfully concentrated sources of enzymes. These are dynamic catalytic substances that have the power to break down the fatty wastes stubbornly clinging to your fat cells and then wash them out of your body. Food enzymes scrub your fat cells and slim them down . . . thus slimming you down, too.

Meet Life-Giving Enzymes

Enzymes are complex proteins that help you to digest food, to absorb nutrients into your bloodstream, and to dispatch nutrients to every part of your body. Enzymes are more than substances. They possess a vital energy essential to the action and activity of every part of your body, for every aspect of life. Without enzymes, there would be no life! This is the power of enzymes in raw foods and juices. You can use this natural power to wash the fat out of your cells.

Enzymes Digest Fat-Calories-Carbohydrates

When you eat foods or drink beverages, your enzymatic system is called into action. If you have an abundance of enzymes, the nutrients in your food and drink are metabolized and washed out of your body. *Problem:* You may be deficient in enzymes. This weakness permits portions of the food you digest, in its incompletely metabolized forms as wastes, to be stored in your adipocytes and give you excess weight. Your cells become fat! So do you!

Quick Ways to Boost Cell-Slimming Enzyme Cleansing

Your goal is to use enzymes to attack the stored-up sludge in your adipose tissue mass. You can do this by releasing more enzymes with improved eating methods. In so doing, you release a high concentration of these inner cleansers to break down and wash out the stubborn fatty wastes clinging to your tissues. Follow these easy programs and wash the fat out of your body almost from the start.

1. *Chew food thoroughly.* In so doing, you release salivary and digestive enzymes that start metabolizing carbohydrates even before it is swallowed. The chewing enzymes help break down wastes and prepare them for elimination more speedily. Salivary ptyalin digests carbohydrates to regulate their storage. Thorough chewing expedites this inner cleansing.

2. *Be cautious about refined sweeteners.* Sugar in any form neutralizes valuable enzymes and renders them weak or helpless. Refined sugar is absorbed speedily with hardly any digestive action. Waste residues cling to your adipocytes and erupt into billowing overweight in no time at all. Refined sweeteners should be avoided!

3. *Do not drown enzymes with liquids at mealtime.* Your enzymes function more vigorously in cell cleansing if they are not drenched with liquids before, during, or immediately after a meal. You will *dilute* these enzymes, weaken their cell-cleansing power. Plan to drink any liquid two hours *before* your meal. Do not drink with meals. Drink two hours *after* your meal. This simple method gives full cell-cleansing power to your enzymes.

4. *Avoid temperature extremes in foods and beverages.* Too hot or too cold foods and beverages either scald or freeze your digestive enzymes. Temperature extremes deactivate vital digestive processes allowing an increase of cellular overload. Whatever you eat or drink should have a comfortable taste temperature. This is healthful for your enzymatic process.

5. *Avoid sharp seasonings.* Salt, pepper, monosodium glutamate, and other volatile seasonings "burn" enzymes and practically destroy them. Sodium, in particular, leaves waste residue behind which then becomes glued to your adipocytes. Worse, they are sponge-like and suck up liquids. You become bloated. You gain excessive weight because of this liquid-engorged salt residue. To avoid, switch to flavorful and mild herbs for cleaner taste and cleaner cells.

6. *Enzymes are found ONLY in raw fruits and vegetables.* When subjected to extremely high or extremely low temperatures, enzymes are weakened and destroyed. While there are certain foods you must cook, you can preserve the potency of enzymes by keeping heat or cold to a minimum. Cook briefly, or, as little as needed to prepare the food. Your goal is to increase your intake of raw fruits and vegetables that are brimming with fat-washing enzymes.

7. *Invigorate enzyme scrubbing action with more exercise.* Keep yourself physically active. You stimulate your metabolism so that enzymes are better able to scrub away calories and fat from your cells. Look at the following chart. See how easy it is to boost enzyme scrubbing with daily fitness.

8. *Bottled juices: how much enzyme power do they have?* Bottled juices are easy to use. But are they beneficial insofar as your cell-scrubbing needs are involved? Look at the label. See if it tells you how much real fruit or vegetable juice it contains. Unless the product says it is all

juice, there is likely to be no reference to the amount of juice in the drink. There is nothing wrong with buying a diluted juice drink, if that's what you want. But if you want pure enzyme-rich juice, the label should say "100 percent juice" or "no water added" or something similar. *Careful:* any drink labeled "cocktail," "beverage," or "juice drink" almost certainly has water and added sugar. Be aware of claims like "100 percent natural." That does NOT mean 100 percent juice. Water, high-fructose corn syrup, and some colors and flavors are considered natural. Although the commercial juicing may deplete some enzymes, the bottled product is reasonably strong in these cell scrubbers.

Of course, with a juicer, you can explore many adventurous flavors not likely to be found on the grocery shelves. *Tip:* Lime brings out unusual flavors in almost all fruits. A tablespoon of lime juice makes any drink an exciting treat. *Example:* Puree banana, mix with a little lime, some salt-free seltzer, a bit of honey, and you have a dynamic cell-scrubbing drink. The same applies for plums, peaches, apples, and many other fruits. Juicers open the doorway to the delightful just-picked taste of fresh fruits and vegetables.

PHYSICAL ACTIVITY
CALORIC EXPENDITURE CHART

Physical Activity	Calories per Hour
Walking 2 m.p.h.	200
3 m.p.h.	270
4 m.p.h.	350
Running	800–1000
Cycling 5 m.p.h.	250
10 m.p.h.	450
14 m.p.h.	700
Horseback riding	
Walk	150
Trot	500
Gallop	200–400

Physical Exercise	Calories per Hour
Gymnastics	200–500
Golf	300
Tennis	400–500
Soccer	550

Physical Exercise	Calories per Hour
Sculling	
50 strokes per min.	420
97 strokes per min.	670
Rowing (peak effort)	1200
Swimming, breast and backstroke	300–650
Crawl (Swimming)	700–900
Squash	600–700
Climbing	700–900
Skiing	600–700
Skating (fast)	300–700
Wrestling	900–1000
Weight Training	500–600
Competitive Body Building	950–1100

Domestic Occupations	Calories per Hour
Sewing	10–30
Writing	20
Sitting at rest	15
Dressing and undressing	30–40
Dishwashing	60
Sweeping or dusting	80–130

Industrial Occupations	Calories per Hour
Tailor	80–130
Shoemaker	80–100
Bookbinder	75–100
Locksmith	150–200
House-painter	150–200
Carpenter	150–200
Joiner	200
Cartwright	200
Riveter	300
Coal miner (av. for shift)	200–400
Stonemason	300–400
Sawyer	400–600

TWENTY-THREE FOODS THAT WASH AWAY YOUR OVERWEIGHT

Here is a list of twenty-three high-enzyme foods that work swiftly at the basic cause of your overweight: washing away the accumulated wastes from your adipocytes. When you eat these foods, your thorough chewing releases enzymes that work speedily to break down the stubborn wastes glued to your adipocytes. You can actually eat your way to lifetime slimness with these cell-cleansing foods.

Suggested Program

Eat several of these foods daily, preferably raw. If cooking is required, steam just long enough until they are tender for chewing. Eat singly or in combination. If seasoning is desired, use a little lemon or lime juice, a sprinkle of apple cider vinegar, or desired herbs.

For powerful super-cell cleansing action, plan to begin *each* meal with several of these cell-washing enzyme vegetables. In this way, they are available for digesting the fat, protein, and carbohydrates from the meal that follows. These enzyme vegetables control or restrict the amount of wastes that are deposited on your adipocytes. In effect, you can eat your way to slimness on this simple and tasty program. *Remember to chew all foods thoroughly.*

asparagus	kale
beans (green)	lettuce
broccoli	mushrooms
brussels sprouts	mustard greens
carrots	parsley
cauliflower	romaine lettuce
celery	squash
chicory	swiss chard
collards	tomato
cucumber	turnip greens
dandelion greens	watercress
escarole	

CASE HISTORY—Sheds 34 Pounds, Shrinks 9 Inches, Within 14 Weeks

Unpleasingly plump Beth Z. waddled instead of walked, spread instead of sat, billowed in whatever she wore. She had a lifetime problem with excess weight. Even worse, it kept increasing. She desperately sought help from a bariatrician (physician who specializes in obesity) who suggested she get to the cause of her problem. Namely, the weighty wastes that clung to her adipocytes. He put her on the cell-scrubbing enzyme program. Beth Z. was told to begin each meal with a selection of some of the listed twenty-three high-enzyme foods. This would set off an immediate enzymatic action that would

(1) wash her fat-filled cells; and (2) metabolize and fully digest eaten foods. This plan would protect against excessive waste clutter in her cells. She was told to control caloric intake, keep physically active, and eliminate refined sugar in any form. Results? The pounds just melted away. Beth Z. saw the scales go down, down, down. Amazed, she was able to shed 34 stubborn pounds, shrink 9 unsightly inches—all within 14 weeks. She soon became a lovely 120-pound woman with a neat and enviable figure. She became *permanently* slim on the enzyme program!

Simple Six-Step Raw Food Plan

The million-dollar health spas of exclusive resorts worldwide charge top dollar to overweight clients from the top echelons of society to follow this simple program. You can do it right at home . . . for free! It consists of a six-step plan you follow on *alternate* days of the week. In between, follow the enzyme scrubbing programs outlined in this chapter and throughout the book. You will discover the fat washing right out of your cells as the scales show less weight, and a tape measure shows inches off. Here is your million-dollar cell-washing plan.

1. *Morning Meal.* Enjoy a plate of fresh fruit in season for breakfast. Select any desired fruit in any favorite combinations. You must chew carefully and thoroughly before you swallow. Eat leisurely. Fruit should be at a comfortable cool temperature, not ice cold.

2. *Mid-Morning Snack.* Drink one or two glasses of either fresh fruit or vegetable juice.

3. *Noon Meal.* Eat a plate of fresh raw vegetables in season. Select any desired combination. Eat leisurely. Chew thoroughly. Vegetables should not be ice cold; keep them at an enzyme-soothing cool temperature.

4. *Mid-Afternoon Snack.* Drink one or two glasses of either fresh fruit or vegetable juice.

5. *Evening Meal.* Prepare a platter of different raw vegetables than those enjoyed earlier. Chew thoroughly.

6. *Late-Evening Snack.* Drink a glass of fresh vegetable juice. Its high mineral treasure is soothing and helps you sleep soundly.

Works While You Sleep

Throughout the day, you have spared your fat-melting digestive system the chore of coping with heavier, cooked foods. Without this interference, enzymes can focus full force on your adipose (fat) cells, dislodging the heavy wastes that are responsible for your obesity. Within an hour after you finish the meal or snack, a treasure of waste-washing enzymes are breaking up cell sludge vigorously, starting the slimming process. This continues throughout the night, while you sleep, when the powerful enzymes do not have to share burdens with heavier and cooked foods.

Next morning, see and feel your weight loss via your mirror and scales. Pounds and inches are falling away because the catalytic enzymes loosened and dissolved the fat from your adipose tissues.

Alternate Days for Raw Food Fast

The million-dollar spas prescribe the preceding dynamic cell-shrinking raw food fast for alternate days. On the other days, eat healthfully and with common sense. But mark your calendar for an entire week, two weeks, or more: put a large *X* through every other day of the week. On each of these days, follow the *Six-Step Raw Food Plan*. When your weight reaches the desired level, you may limit the plan to one or two days a week. Spa specialists suggest a "maintenance" program of one fast day every ten days. It keeps your catalytic enzymes in tiptop shape as they keep your cells in well-scrubbed slim shape, too.

CASE HISTORY—**From "Fat" to "Slim" in One Weekend**

When Jeff X's insurance company wanted to cancel his policy because of his increasing corpulence, he needed to act swiftly. The company physician, who studied the miraculous weight-losing programs of health spas, told Jeff X. to follow a three-day weekend raw food program. Anxious to shed his undesirable weight, Jeff X. tried the regimen. It was pleasing because he liked to "chew on something" while dieting. Other diets left him unsatisfied, but chewing raw fruits and vegetables did give him the pleasure he rightfully deserved. Almost at once, his adipose cells started to shrink. Within two days the pounds and inches melted away. When he finished the weekend, he had shed so much unwanted weight, he was dubbed "Slim" (he used to be called "Fat" behind his back) and was accepted for insurance renewal. It took just one weekend for this "miracle" to happen.

TWO SIMPLE STEPS THAT PROTECT AGAINST CELLULAR OVERWEIGHT

Why Are Cells Overloaded?

Briefly, when you consume calories from fats, proteins, and carbohydrates, these substances are transformed into *adenosine triphosphate* (ATP). This waste product is then deposited in your cells if not burned off at the time of intake. Therefore, your cells become overweight because of the stored-up ATP.

Can You Reduce Cells?

Your body must provide enzymatic energy that will enter the cells and dislodge the ATP waste, thereby starting cellular slimming. Enzymes are the substances needed to bring about this melting away of ATP wastes from your cells. To provide cell-slimming enzymes that "attack" the stubborn ATP clumps, follow these two simple steps:

1. Begin each meal with a raw vegetable platter. *Inner Cleansing Benefit:* Carefully chewed vegetables provide both food and digestive enzymes, which actually "shower" your cells and wash away the ATP clumps.
2. Finish each meal with a raw fruit platter. *Inner Cleansing Benefit:* Ingested foods, with their high caloric waste deposition, will not be allowed to remain when fruit enzymes drive forth to uproot and wash them out of your system right after the meal.

Easy, Effective, Enzymatic

This easy change is effective quickly via the enzymatic dispatchers that work right on the spot to nip cellular overweight in the bud.

CASE HISTORY—**Eats and Loses Weight with Two-Step Plan**

Years of cellular overloading made Judy O'H. "hopelessly" fat. Then a nutrition counselor suggested she follow the preceding two-step plan to boost release of cell-slimming enzymes. Judy O'H. cut down on size of portions and fats, but still ate wholesomely with just these simple changes: a raw vegetable platter before a meal to release the inner cleansing enzymes and a raw fruit platter after a meal to double enzymatic catalytic action upon ingested food. Result? She could eat and still shrink down her weight almost from the start. Over 40 pounds "disappeared" on this cell-washing plan. And the joy of it was that Judy O'H. could still eat most of her favorite foods . . . as long as she used the vegetable-fruit program. It was the most delicious reducing program she ever followed, and it worked!

SAY "NO" TO THESE WASTE CAUSING FOODS

Put the red "stop" light on these danger foods. They add cement-like sludge to your adipose cells and harden them to such a thickness, it would require

Herculean enzymes to get them off. Avoid this problem by avoiding these waste-causing foods:

soft drinks and sodas	cookies	fried foods
chocolate	cakes	sweetened cereals
candy	pies	sweetened fruit or vegetable drinks
jellies	sugar	bacon/fatty meats
jams	pretzels	sausages
ice cream	potato chips	alcoholic drinks
doughnuts	gravies	salt

In Brief: Anything that contains either sugar or salt is a "no-no." These are dangerous sources of thick sludge on your cells. Avoid such waste-causing foods and you avoid cellular overload and body overweight.

You can wash the weight right out of your cells by eating the right foods and drinking healthy beverages and avoiding the wrong ones. You'll discover you can actually eat your way to a slim-trim figure and a more youthful body.

--------------------------- *HIGHLIGHTS* ---------------------------

1. *Cellular overload, the real root cause of overweight, can be conquered with the intake of raw food enzymes.*

2. *Boost cell-slimming enzyme release with the basic eight-step plan.*

3. *Eat freely of the twenty-three foods that actually wash away your overweight.*

4. *Beth Z. shed 45 pounds and shrank 9 inches within 14 weeks by eating a variety of these twenty-three foods, in any desired combination or quantity. You, too, can achieve the same results by eating all you want of such cell-scrubbing foods.*

5. *The million-dollar health spas offer a six-step raw food plan that works miracles in stimulating dramatic weight loss.*

6. *Jeff X. went from "fat" to "slim" in one weekend on the easy raw food plan.*

7. *Two simple remedies used by Judy O'H. gave her dramatic weight loss.*

Chapter 7

FREE YOURSELF FROM ALLERGIES WITH CELLULAR WASHING

With each breath you take, you deposit an overwhelming amount of toxic pollutants on the millions of cells and tissues that make up your respiratory organs. These waste particles need to be washed out constantly so that oxygen exchange can take place freely. But in a polluted environment, together with the eating of chemically treated foods, toxic wastes overwhelm the usual self-cleaning process and respiratory pollution takes hold to cause allergies.

BODY POLLUTION TRIGGERS ALLERGIES

As toxic wastes accumulate, they cause the lining membranes of your bronchial tubes to swell. Internal body pollution causes contraction of the surrounding musculature and plugs the tubes by depositing more and more waste particles. Thick mucus is a major form of lung pollution. If these wastes are allowed to accumulate, they predispose toward problems of asthma, serious coughs, extreme dust sensitivities, seasonal allergies (hay fever, for example), and frightening shortness of breath. This last-named problem can cause such an oxygen deficiency that cardiovascular distress may strike. So you can see that toxic wastes allowed to stick to your bronchial tubes can shorten the very breath of life!

Check Your Own Breathing Problem

Are there times when you gasp for air? Even if you climb a small staircase, does it leave you breathless? You may have trouble *exhaling,* more so than *inhaling.* What's the difference? Exhalation difficulties tell you that the air passages of your bronchi have become clogged with waste particles and constricted with toxic-like mucus, thus squeezing the passages. This makes it hard for you to breathe *out*. It is a sign that your breathing apparatus has become overloaded with toxic wastes. You need to start cellular washing so you can say goodbye to the choking, sputtering, desperate need for precious air. You can follow these methods of inner cleansing in the privacy of your home. They work swiftly and effectively to help you get rid of allergy-causing wastes.

ONE-DAY JUICE FAST = FREEDOM FROM ALLERGIES

The accumulated glue-like sludge that has fastened to your bronchial tubes needs to be jarred loose and eliminated so you can free yourself from this irritation. This can be done through the powerful detoxifying powers of *lemon juice*.

The high concentration of bioflavonoids as well as vitamin C, enzymes, and natural fruit acids, have the power to dislodge, break down, and wash away toxic wastes that have glued themselves to your lungs.

How to Prepare

In a glass of freshly boiled water, squeeze the juice of one or two fresh lemons. Add a dab of honey, if desired. Stir slowly. When tepid, drink this lung-cleansing lemonade.

How Much to Drink

Throughout the day, take no other foods or beverages (except water). Instead, drink up to six or eight glasses of this lemon juice cleanser. This is a powerful and effective lung-washing juice fast.

Cleanses Lungs, Washes Cells

The lemon juice cleanser is rich in vigorous enzymes that break down accumulated wastes; the natural vitamin C helps rebuild the collagen and cellular walls to strengthen them against the onslaught of continuous pollution you inhale with every breath . . . right at this minute! Your lungs become cleansed. Your cells are washed and restored. Sparkling clean, you are now able to breathe more healthfully.

Simple Program

Depending upon the severity of your lung pollution, you should plan on having this one-day lemon juice fast every seven days. As your bronchial tubes become cleansed, as the irritating debris is scrubbed away and your breathing is refreshingly easier, you may reduce the frequency of the lemon juice fast. Thereafter, schedule this cell-washing fast twice a month for lifetime freedom from allergic distress.

CASE HISTORY—**Conquers Hopeless Asthma in Two Days with Juice Fast**

A victim of childhood asthma, Alma DeB. was told that her case was "hopeless" and she would have to live with her breathing problem. She chose, instead, to find a way to live without this choking affliction. A naturopathic physician discovered via an examination that her bronchial tubes were covered with accumulated glue-like wastes. They so irritated her fragile respiratory cells that any particle inhaled would bring on an asthmatic attack.

Alma DeB. was told to go on a two-day lemon juice fast. She was to avoid all other foods and beverages. Instead, take up to eight glasses of this lemon juice drink. *Reason:* the lemon substances would work without interference from other consumed foods or liquids. Almost at once, Alma DeB. was able to breathe more easily. By the middle of the second day the lemon juice had so cleansed her bronchial tubes that she could breathe deeply with welcome comfort. By the end of the second day, she had fully recovered. Thereafter, she never again had an asthma attack. To be on the safe side, she cleans her bronchial cells and tissues with a lemon juice fasting program once every ten days. It helps her say "goodbye forever" to her asthma allergy attacks.

ASTHMA—WHY DOES IT HAPPEN?

Asthma is a noncontagious allergy of the lungs, specifically the bronchial tubes. These are the tubes that carry air from the mouth to the air sacs in the lungs. In asthma, these tubes are obstructed. This obstruction is due to: (1) swelling of the inside lining of the tubes; (2) contraction (squeezing down) of the muscles surrounding the tubes thus reducing their diameter; (3) excessive mucus production which often hardens wastes and toxic debris within the tubes producing plugs.

Inner Culprit Is Found

Why does it happen? Substances called *leukotrienes* are among the chief culprits in a variety of allergic reactions. Leukotrienes tighten air passages in the lungs and increase mucus-waste production in the nose. Leukotrienes are made in the body through a complex chemical process that involves inhaled pollutants that form these glue-like irritants.

DANGER: An overwhelming assault of leukotrienes will make you hypersensitive to allergens such as pollens, molds, dust, and animal danders. You may also develop hay fever.

What Is Hay Fever?

Also known as allergic rhinitis, hay fever is caused primarily by pollens from ragweed and certain grasses and trees. They are usually seasonal and windborne. You inhale these sticky and heavy pollens, and the leukotrienes start to choke your breathing apparatus. The cells lining your nose, eyes, and air passages release *histamine,* a complex chemical substance, to fight the irritation. You have an excess of histamine and you react with swollen nasal passages, sensitive membranes, itching and watery eyes, constant sneezing. This condition often lasts until the end of the particular seasonal pollen. (See accompanying chart.)

SEASONAL HAY FEVER

	East and Midwest	South and South Central	West
SPRING	Tree pollen: oak, sycamore, birch	Tree pollen	Tree pollen
SUMMER	Grass pollen: blue-grass, redtop	Grass pollen	Grass pollen
FALL	Ragweed pollen In August and Sept. a quarter of a million tons of pollen blow through the Midwest.	Grass pollen Ragweed pollen	Tumbleweed and sage pollen
WINTER		Tree pollen Grass pollen	Tumbleweed and sage pollen
YEAR-ROUND	Mold spores on soil and vegetation are spread from April through November and trigger severe allergic reactions. Frost does not kill them.	In central Florida the ragweed seasons runs from June to November.	Because of lower ragweed pollen levels and higher elevations, the area in general offers sufferers a respite from seasonal allergies. Mold spores decrease at high altitudes and in dry areas.

Source: the American Academy of Allergy and Immunology

Nutritional Cleansers

To ease the choking of the leukotrienes and histamine, several nutrients are helpful. These are:

Vitamin B₆. It helps increase your resistance to pollutants; this vitamin also helps take the sting out of the leukotrienes and minimizes the assault of the histamine. About 100 milligrams daily is useful.

Vitamin C. It reduces the sensitivity that asthmatics have to air pollutants. It also helps reduce bronchial spasms. Vitamin C reduces sensitivity to pollutants in the air and prevents hurtful throat spasms. About 2000 milligrams daily boosts this resistance.

Magnesium. It is needed for proper muscle relaxation. Asthma is often felt as a violent muscle spasm in the region of chest and throat. This mineral is needed for inner cleansing. About 400 milligrams daily is important in your inner cleansing of allergies.

TEN STEPS TO EASE ALLERGIC REACTIONS

Arthur Lubitz, M.D., a specialist in allergies, assistant clinical instructor at New York Medical College, offers these lung-sparing suggestions:

1. Become a pollen expert. Learn when and where pollens are most prevalent. A simplified chart of where and when certain pollens thrive is important. But never guess about the source of your symptoms and see a qualified allergist.

2. Chill out your allergies. Air-conditioning is one of the best ways to lessen allergen exposure. Central systems work best. Keep air-conditioning set at the highest comfortable setting—not lower than 70°. If you're not at home, don't leave your set on, since it tends to pull in daytime pollen. And be sure to clean your air filter or wash it at least once a month.

3. Catch a sea breeze. Wind blowing in from the ocean is refreshing as long as it doesn't pass over a land mass before reaching you. Air blowing out to sea is some of the most allergen-laden. Beach weather—a hot sun and a strong breeze will give you a schnozola full of allergies.

4. Take advantage of summer showers since they wash pollen out of the air. However, if you're mold-allergic, your symptoms may be worse right after several days of showers because humidity promotes mold growth.

5. Become a tea-totaller. Alcoholic beverages increase the severity of allergic reactions in some people, especially when the air is thick with allergens. Wine and beer are the worst offenders.

6. You may love watermelon, but chances are it doesn't love you. People allergic to ragweed often cross-react with a variety of botanically similar species. These include watermelon and mango.

7. You may not be bugged by bugs, but that insecticide might set you scratching. Pyrethrum, an alternative to chemical-based bug killers which protects the environment, is made from crushed chrysanthemums and can make hay fever victims miserable.

8. If you're allergy prone, don't dive or swim underwater. Swelling inside the ears is a fairly common allergic reaction. The stress and pressure changes that accompany diving into the water can greatly aggravate ears that pop or feel plugged to allergen exposure.

9. Whether or not you're lactose intolerant (allergic to dairy products), if you are prone to allergies, then cut down on dairy foods.

10. Hazardous materials frequently found in the manufacture of products commonly found in our work and home environments are threatening. "Sick Building Syndrome" is the term used to describe the potentially lethal effect of certain chemicals frequently used in the manufacture of products common to our home and workplace. For instance, *isocyanate,* a chemical used in the manufacture of polyurethane foam (found in seat cushions, carton packaging, and refrigerator insulation) is believed to have led to a dramatic increase in respiratory ills such as asthma.

"When all is said and done, the greatest threat to asthmatics is the undiagnosed, untreated allergies which cause their respiratory ills," says Dr. Arthur Lubitz. "There are a myriad of tests now utilized by allergists from the traditional skin prick test, to provocation tests, to the radio allergosorbent test (RAST), a blood test used in measuring the amount of immunoglobulin E antibody that reacts to specific allergens."[16]

TIPS TO TAME SPRING ALLERGIES

With some planning, you can avoid most potential allergens that will deposit sludge on your breathing apparatus. Here's how:

• Avoid staying outdoors between 4:00 A.M. and 10:00 A.M. when pollen levels are highest.

- Keep windows closed in your home as well as in your car while driving.
- Keep cool—but not too cold, because "superfreezing" indoor temperatures may aggravate allergy symptoms. Ten degrees cooler than outside is ideal. Be sure to keep air conditioners and humidifiers scrupulously clean or you may end up blowing allergens around your home.
- Wear glasses or sunglasses outdoors to protect your eyes from pollen.
- Keep your lawn mowed short—most clipped grasses can't bloom, which is what releases pollen spores. Wear a mask while you are mowing your lawn or gardening.
- Shower and shampoo if you think you've been exposed to pollen. Wash your hands thoroughly and rinse your eyes with warm water every time you come indoors.
- Dry clothing and bedding inside, or in a dryer, rather than outdoors where they will collect pollen.
- Use allergen-proof casings for pillows, mattresses, and box springs. Vacuum all casings frequently. Store nothing under the bed.
- Avoid rugs or carpets in your house; use only wood or linoleum flooring.
- Avoid pets altogether, or at least restrict pets to certain rooms—never the bedroom.
- Avoid alcoholic beverages; they contribute to swelling of blood vessels in nasal passages. Avoid cigarette smoke whenever you can, and certainly don't smoke yourself.
- Don't grow too many indoor plants; wet dirt causes molds to form.

CLEAN UP YOUR LIFESTYLE AND CLEAN UP YOUR BREATHING ORGANS

Constant Waste Dumping

Air pollution, cigarette smoke, and crowded living and working conditions all deposit wastes upon your breathing organs. You inhale close to 3000 gallons of air per day. This polluted air causes a constant waste dumping on your lungs. These toxic pollutants include carbon dioxide, carbon monoxide, hydrogen sulfide, hydrocarbons from auto exhausts, asbestos, carbon particulates, and rubber compounds. The list is endless. These airborne pollutants actually "choke" your breathing organs.

Little Chance of Escape

Rural areas do have less pollutants but still are not as safe as you would wish them to be. Winds carry wastes from industrial and crowded areas for hundreds of miles from the original source. Country living offers little escape from the constant assault of waste-accumulating pollutants.

Build Resistance at Home

The answer here is to build within yourself as much resistance to lung pollution as possible. You can begin right at home. By cleaning your home lifestyle, you help clean your breathing organs. You can enjoy more than allergy freedom; you can have a healthier and longer lifetime. Start today to bring about these changes at home:

1. Remove everything that gives off unpleasant odors. Keep them out of inhalation range until absolutely needed for use and then use only in a ventilated area. Pollution-causing items include furniture polishes, window and oven cleaners, insecticides, cosmetics, hair sprays, nail polish and remover, paint in any form, commercial glues, and medications. All give off fumes that seep through containers and right into your lungs. Out of scent . . . out of your lungs.

2. Have your automatic stove pilot light turned off, professionally, if need be. It is a constant source of indoor pollution and gas seepage. Keep gas use to an absolute minimum, whether at the stove or dryer or heater.

3. Check food wrappings carefully. Caution: Plastic containers (whether cardboard-like or flexible) are heat-sealed onto the food. Pollutants leach out and contaminate the food. Whenever possible, opt for fresh, unpackaged foods as much as you can. Glass enclosed products are good, too.

4. If you want to keep clean and look good then use more natural products. Use ordinary baking soda (with or without a pinch of salt) as a dentifrice and mouth wash. Men, try an electric razor. For an astringent, use ordinary ice water. Use baby soaps and baby shampoos because they're much milder and less polluting than the adult variety. Replace any plastic containers with glass—even cardboard is preferable to plastic.

5. Clothing should be washed in a detergent-free biodegradable washing soda or soap. Otherwise, chemicals in washing materials and rinses

cling to the garments and then penetrate your pores. *Simple Test:* Sprinkle a few drops of water on a ready-to-wear garment. If the water penetrates through, the garment is healthy to wear. If it remains on top, the garment is chemically polluted and you would do well to avoid its use. *Tip:* Read garment labels. Select items that are made from natural fibers (cotton and wool, for example), without any synthetics.

6. Restrict or eliminate any use of rubber. That includes plastic foam. Bedding should be as natural as possible. Sheets, pillow cases, blankets should all be of a natural material. Avoid the use of polyester for bedding since the warmth of your body will release its hydrocarbons which then enter your open pores to create internal pollution. CAUTION: Avoid use of an electric blanket. Yes, it is warm, but its wires are sealed in plastic and when heated will give off an invisible vapor that enters your body. Instead, garb yourself in woolen nightclothes.

7. Cookwear should be stainless steel, cast iron, or copper, *not* aluminum. Heating aluminum gives off noxious waste-laden fumes. Avoid frying because it forms tars on foods and also leads to indoor pollution.

8. Wash pots and dishes with tap water and any soap that is detergent-free or biodegradable. Use the same type of washing soda as you do for clothing. Rinse thoroughly. CAUTION: Do not use paper towels because they are coated with chemicals and various chlorine bleaches. Remember to *avoid* plastics of any sort, and that includes cookwear and serving wear, too.

9. Check all of your heating systems and exhaust fans. In just one hour (at 350° F.) your gas oven can give off concentrations of carbon monoxide and nitrogen dioxide that can trigger an allergic attack. Make certain your exhaust fans work perfectly. [Always keep windows open to let fumes escape.]

10. Keep your living and working quarters clean and dry. Avoid dampness—it promotes growth of molds and spores that are inhaled and can coat your lungs until you develop allergic attacks.

Remember, such toxic wastes can penetrate your mucous membranes, be swallowed, and then be taken up via your gastrointestinal tract, increasing levels of body pollution. Make these basic adjustments in your lifestyle. You will be able to breathe better. Longer, too!

ASTHMA CHECKLIST

☑ Do not smoke. Avoid areas where others are smoking.

☑ Keep your apartment as dust-free as you can: dust and vacuum often; avoid shag rugs; wash bedding and curtains often in hot water.

☑ If possible, do not keep pets. Otherwise, keep the pet out of the asthma patient's bedroom.

☑ Keep your home as free of cockroaches as possible. Store food properly and use roach-killing products.

☑ Keep bathrooms and basements well-ventilated to prevent mold growth.

☑ Avoid heavy exercise in cold, dry weather. If aspirin sets off your asthma, be sure to read labels of over-the-counter medicines which may contain aspirin.

☑ Use an air conditioner when possible in the summer, especially when pollution is bad.

Checklist provided by Fisons Corporation

QUICK HELP FOR ALLERGIC SYMPTOMS

For quick help, try some of these natural remedies:

- *Bronchial Infections.* Eat several raw garlic cloves for their strong antibiotic power.
- *Fluid-Mucus Pollution in Lungs and Air Passages.* For swift inner cleansing of this sludge, drink a cup of hot horehound tea with a squeeze of lemon or lime. Drink three to four cups throughout the day.
- *Hacking Cough Spasms.* Drink a cup of coltsfoot tea—an infusion of the leaves and flowers soothe the air passages, heal tissue, and scrub the delicate mucous membranes.
- *Choking Difficulties.* Cowslip flower syrup or a cup of tea made from the roots (available from an herbalist), is very soothing to ease spasms and clear mucus.
- *Expectorant.* Aniseed tea has a natural expectorant action and works like a chemicalized cough mixture except that it boosts inner cleansing of the bronchial tubes.
- *Hay Fever.* A cup of goldenrod tea relieves your irritated mucous membranes. Several cups throughout the day minimize the pollution

effects. Other herbal teas that soothe the distress include: hyssop, lavender, thyme, marjoram. Mix and match.

- *Irritated Eyes.* Soak a clean cloth in witch hazel diluted in four parts boiled water. Apply as a cold compress to soothe your eyes. To eliminate excess mucus, try a cup of hot mullein flower tea. To reduce redness, try eyebright tea.

Drink several cups of these herbal teas throughout the day. You may build immunity to these symptoms by drinking these teas as a regular beverage all year long. Much better than coffee or commercial tea that are laced with caffeine and chemicals!

ALTERNATE NOSTRIL BREATHING TECHNIQUE FOR INTERNAL CLEANSING

Your Nose: The Body's Air-Conditioner

The mucous membranes of your nasal cavities have the ability to promote body air conditioning. Inhalation programs bring about a freer exchange of air to promote a more vigorous dislodging and subsequent removal of accumulated pollutants.

The suction used during a helpful remedy known as "alternate nostril breathing" helps draw pollutants out of your respiratory tract and thereby creates an important cleansing reaction. This can be easily done at home or anywhere else you have five minutes to spare. It helps decongest your respiratory organs so you can breathe with refreshing comfort.

Asthma, Sensitivities, Coughs Are Relieved

This "alternate nostril breathing" program discharges enough irritants to give you speedy relief from asthmatic attacks, sensitivities to dust, and stubborn coughs. Plan to use this remedy (1) whenever you feel a breathing problem threatening to take hold; and (2) as a maintenance program, at least once or twice each day. Simply follow this four-step program:

1. Breathe in through both sides of your nose. Breathe out through one side, closing your other nostril with your finger.
2. Breathe in and out through the same side, closing the other side with your finger.
3 Breathe in through the side that is less blocked. Breathe out through the other side, closing the unused nostril with your finger.

4. If both sides are blocked, breathe in through your mouth and out through one side of your nose as forcibly as necessary. As soon as one side of your nose opens sufficiently to allow it, then breathe in through the open side. Stop the mouth breathing.

Suggestion: Just five minutes of this "alternate nostril breathing" method each day will help control the inner pollutant level and more important, help wash out those irritating wastes. You'll find it easier and more refreshing as you breathe better. This method also gives you greater immunity to future allergic problems. Over a period of time, allergies will be washed away!

CASE HISTORY—Breathes Free and Overcomes Allergies in Five Days

Construction engineer Morton Y.S. would suffer from choked breath when climbing only a few steps. On the job site, he turned blue, gasped for air, and sputtered with his tongue hanging out after walking a short distance. His condition so worsened that a slight bit of dust or pollution gave him a stuffed nose in minutes. This almost asphyxiated him. Such a disability threatened his career. The company respiratory specialist suggested he help wash away the breath-choking pollution with the "alternate nostril breathing" method. Morton Y.S. took frequent "breathing breaks" as he called them. Almost four times daily, he would use the method. Within five days, he could breathe freely. He overcame his allergies. Now, he can work (and breathe) with the vigor of a healthy youngster!

WHISTLE YOUR WAY TO CLEANER LUNGS

Just as your normal breathing power sucks in pollution and deposits stubborn grime upon your lungs, so can the reverse method help remove these allergy-causing wastes. You can do this with a very easy trick—*whistling*.

Twenty-five–Cent Whistle = Million-Dollar Throat

Get yourself a whistle at any toy store. It costs about 25 cents or even less. Whenever you are out of earshot, just whistle! The forceful blowing will vacuum out your lungs. Toxic wastes and dirt will be uprooted and washed out. *Suggestion:* To silence the whistle, remove the little pit-like nuggets.

Using a whistle (whether silent or chirping) requires you to *pucker* your lips. This improves the vacuum cleaner effect and is more vigorous in uprooting and casting out cell-eroding wastes. Whistle as often as possible for speedy and refreshing lung cleansing.

An allergic reaction is an unhealthy response to accumulated wastes that have entered your body. Pollens, dust, a whiff of exhaust from a car, the scent of perfume or of almost any synthetic compound can cause a reaction. A toxin can be as insidious as the invisible asbestos dust seeping from your walls, or fumes from almost any source. Toxins have also been known to trigger autoimmune reactions in which your body reacts against its own tissue, resulting in many illnesses. Do not disregard them. Repeated and un-treated toxic exposures will inevitably lead to some kind of serious illness. Begin inner cleansing promptly.

The breath of life should be exactly that—life-giving. Protect your body against cellular congestion and the choking agony of allergic attacks with these cleansing programs. Breathing will then provide refreshing nour-ishment and youthful vigor. You will then be able to say goodbye forever to so-called "hopeless" allergies.

———————————— *HIGHLIGHTS* ————————————

1. *Nip lung congestion in the bud with a one-day lemon juice fast. It washes away accumulated debris and helps you breathe better.*

2. *Alma DeB. conquered hopeless asthma in two days with the lemon juice fast.*

3. *A noted allergist offers a set of steps to ease/erase problems of asthma, hay fever and general sensitivity to toxins.*

4. *You can tame spring allergies with the set of cleansing tips.*

5. *Refresh your home—cast out indoor pollution to cast out body pollution.*

6. *Herbal remedies are "natural medicines" for breathing problems.*

7. *Air-condition your body with "alternate nostril breathing" tech-niques.*

8. *Morton Y.S. overcame allergies in five days with a simple breathing remedy.*

9. *Whistling (quietly, please) is a simple and fun way to clean your lungs and protect against allergies.*

Chapter 8

HOW TO SUPERCHARGE YOUR HEART WITH YOUTHFUL POWER . . . WHILE YOU SLEEP!

Cleanse your heart while you sleep and awaken with a feeling of renewed vitality. With the use of stimulating foods and programs you perform during the day, the inner cleansing process will wash away debris from your heart and arteries throughout the night. A catalytic reaction metabolizes and removes wastes to promote inner detoxification. When you wake up, you'll have a clean heart—and a healthier life.

CAUTION: TOXEMIA CAUSES HEART DISTRESS

To understand how internal washing benefits your heart while you sleep, it is helpful to see how toxemia is a threat to cardiac (and total body) health. You will then see how vital it is for you to follow the simple but powerfully effective detoxification programs to bring about "heart washing."

Sneaky Sludge Threatens Heart Health

Accumulated wastes are "sneaky" because they cling together to form heart-threatening sludge over a period of time, without your awareness. These wastes, from eating wrong foods and from environmental pollution, cling to your arteries. Gradually, the inner walls of your arteries become thickened and misshapen with more and more deposits of these fatty wastes. Called *atheromata,* these fatty wastes accumulate sneakily in your blood vessels. If not washed out, they block the blood vessels and threaten cardiovascular trouble. The sludge may cause an occlusion (blockage) or serious arteriosclerosis of the blood vessels in your brain.

The key to protection against these disabling penalties of accumulated sludge is following a simple, effective inner cleansing program as early as possible.

INTERNAL WASHING PROTECTS AGAINST HEART ATTACK

By keeping your heart cleansed, you protect it against the threat of an attack. How is this possible? If fatty sludge is left to accumulate, your two most important blood vessels, the right and left coronary arteries which begin at the base of the aorta (large artery that carries blood from your heart throughout your body), become blocked with fatty waste deposits.

This blockage denies the heart muscle its needed oxygen and nutrients. The heart muscle actually dies! This is one result of the sludge problem. The dead heart muscle is surrounded by an area of acute injury and an area of temporary injury or waste-causing inflammation called an *infarction*. This injured area weakens the heart, which loses some of its effectiveness as a pump because there is less muscle to contract and force blood out.

Sludge Pile-Up Worsens Problem

As more and more wastes pile up, they raise blood pressure and cause an irregular heart rate. The sludge chokes your body's oxygen-carrying abilities, denying your heart its much-needed supply of the "breath of life." The buildup of carbon monoxide in the blood heightens the risk of clots that could block the heart. As sludge mounts up, the heart becomes so choked, it is at high risk of a heart attack. You need to cast out wastes! Your first step is through nutritional improvement. Foods can clean your heart!

WASTE-FORMING VS. WASTE-CLEANING FOODS

We can divide foods into two groups: one group leads to waste formation; the other group leads to waste cleaning. Plan your eating program to cut down on the waste-forming foods and boost intake of waste-cleaning foods. Here are simple guidelines to help you clean your heart:

1. Limit waste-forming foods such as: dairy foods that contain fat; fatty meats such as beef, pork, lamb; oil-packed foods (mayonnaise or salad dressing); hydrogenated products (shortening, margarine); egg yolks; sugar, salt, and products made with these flavorings; and chemically treated foods.

2. Increase waste-cleaning foods such as: fresh fruits and vegetables in any variety and quantity, their fresh juices, foods made with whole

grains, very lean animal foods, legumes, egg whites, and fat-free dairy products.

Watch for "Hidden" Fatty Wastes That Clog Your Heart

These include the butter or margarine on your bread and vegetables, the oil used to fry foods, the chunks of white fat on meat (it should be trimmed off). But that's not all: many foods contain fatty wastes you cannot see: whole milk, hard cheese, ice cream, and "marbled" meats. Eliminate or restrict intake of these fatty-waste foods, and you can control sludge accumulation that threatens to choke the life out of your heart.

POTASSIUM—POWERFUL HEART CLEANSER

People taking blood pressure medicines know their doctors keep a careful watch on their potassium levels. Some drugs make the body excrete much of this valuable mineral. Potassium is a vital mineral that is essential for muscle contractions. The most significant muscle, your heart, depends on potassium for inner cleansing so that it can perform with regularity.

Potassium Protects Against Stroke

Potassium is an *electrolyte,* a substance that conducts an electrical charge. It plays an important role in the transmission of nerve impulses for muscle contraction. In particular, it can build immunity against life-threatening stroke.

DANGER: Stroke is the tornado of cardiovascular disease—feared by many, it hits speedily and unexpectedly, leaving survivors and their families in upheaval. The third leading cause of death, stroke often entails a slow struggle to regain speech and movement capabilities for those who do survive. Nearly two out of three stroke survivors may be permanently disabled afterward.

Potassium brings about an important mineral balance in your cells, primarily involving sodium levels. Potassium cleans out excess sodium and restores tranquility to your cells, establishing a ratio that can save your heart—and life.

Cleansing Potassium Creates Balance in Cells

Sodium and potassium atoms each have an electrical charge attached to them. If you have too much sodium sludge and not enough cleansing potassium in the cells surrounding your arteries, an electrical imbalance strikes. This leads to sodium overload. The arteries clamp down too forcibly when they contract. The result is elevated blood pressure, strain on artery walls, slowing of blood flow to some smaller arteries. Sodium sludge chokes circulation. There is risk of an artery clot that could choke off blood to the heart or brain. You could become the victim of a stroke and/or heart attack.

Potassium Cleanses Cells

This heart-scrubbing mineral regulates the amount of pressure-boosting sodium in cells. Your cells do need some sodium to function. But if sodium is allowed to accumulate excessively inside your cells, there is an increase in blood pressure and risk of heart trouble. Accumulated sludge weakens your cell walls; your heart becomes choked for oxygen. You need potassium to boost inner cleansing to keep sodium moving out of your cells.

Where to Get Cleansing Potassium

Easy . . . tasty. The Food and Nutrition Board of the National Academy of Sciences-National Research Council estimates that adults need 1875 to 5625 milligrams of potassium daily. If this sounds like a lot, be aware that much is eliminated through perspiration. Diuretics, diarrhea, alcohol, excessive urination, increased physical activity all drain out this mineral. So add certain foods to be sure your heart has enough of this cleansing potassium.

Sources: A banana has 450 milligrams; 10 dried apricot halves have 482 milligrams; a cup of fresh cantaloupe has 494. Try low-fat dairy foods such as a cup of milk for 350 milligrams or yogurt for 500 milligrams. Use lots of sprouts, seeds, and nuts. They are potassium gold mines. It's easy to enjoy potassium in salad bowl combinations that are juicy, good to look at, crunchy, and delicious to provide lots of heart-cleansing and pep-up nutrients. Try the following:

- Chopped apples, cabbage, celery, fresh or dried mint, sunflower seeds, assorted sprouts.
- Grated cauliflower on romaine lettuce, thinly sliced carrots, Jerusalem artichokes, pumpkin seeds, mung bean sprouts.
- Diced or sliced red cabbage, pineapple wedges, sliced squash, sesame seeds, lentil sprouts, watercress.
- Chopped apples and walnut meats; moisten with a bit of fruit juice and a dusting of cinnamon. Serve on favorite bean sprouts and a bed of chopped greens.

Heart-Cleansing Potassium Broth

1 cup chopped celery (leaves included)
1 cup grated carrots
1 tablespoon brewer's or nutritional yeast
1 tablespoon chopped watercress
1 quart water
1 cup salt-free or reduced-sodium tomato juice
1 teaspoon herbal seasonings
1 teaspoon honey

In a soup kettle, combine all vegetables and water. Cover and cook slowly for half an hour. Add tomato juice, seasonings, honey. Steam for five more minutes. Let cool—and then enjoy as a soup-like broth with whole grain bread.

Heart-Cleansing Potassium Broth is a powerhouse of nutrients that scrub your cells clean, help balance sodium levels, and protect against sludge-induced strokes or heart attacks.

CLEANSE YOUR HEART WHILE YOU SLEEP

During the day, for your scheduled meals, plan to take in a variety of fresh fruits and vegetables, whole grains, legumes, and low-fat or non-fat dairy products. Enjoy several glasses of fresh fruit and vegetable juices.

Catalytic Reaction Works Overnight

The rich concentration of catalytic enzymes in raw foods are stimulated by the invigorating vitamins and minerals in the same produce. These enzymes dislodge and break down the accumulated deposits that would otherwise cling stubbornly to the inner walls of your arteries. The enzymes initiate a thermal cauterization reaction wherein they actually melt away the porridge-like toxic waste accumulation and prepare the sludge for elimination. This works while you sleep!

CASE HISTORY—From "Choked Breath" to "Vitality" Within 48 Hours

Henry O'H. was a sedentary bookkeeper. This inactivity surely contributed to his toxic waste overload. He would consume large amounts of the waste-forming foods that dumped excessive amounts of sludge throughout his cardiovascular system. He had "choked breath" and a pale skin. At times, his heart pounded so furiously, he feared it would burst. An exam by his cardiologist revealed this dangerous toxemia. He needed quick relief. Henry also complained of feeling sluggish and exhausted. This was traced to his "choked" oxygen supply. He needed to detoxify his heart without delay. He was told to devote three days a week to the "waste-cleaning" foods. The remaining four days included his usual diet, but fats, salt, sugar, and artificial ingredients were taboo. Henry O'H. immediately started this easy detoxification program. Every day, he enjoyed the Heart-Cleansing Potassium Broth. "For backup," he would say. *Results:* Almost overnight, the deposits were loosened. They could be easily washed out of his body. Within 48 hours, he was able to breath healthfully. He had rejuvenated vitality, too. His skin glowed. He no longer had the "choking" sensations. Now he realized that a clean heart had given him a clean body and a more youthful source of energy—possible through the cleansing foods.

GARLIC: AMAZING HEART CLEANSER

This potent vegetable has the amazing power to uproot and cast out fatty wastes that threaten the health of your heart—and your entire body.

Secret of Garlic's Heart-Cleansing Power

Garlic has a rich concentration of allicin. This is an active sulfur-containing substance that is transformed by your metabolism into a unique sludge-washing agent called diallyldisulfide. Your enzymatic system uses this agent to chip away, break down, melt, and actually dissolve the gluey wastes that stubbornly cling to your cardiovascular system. This is the astonishing secret of garlic's heart-cleansing power.

Controls Cholesterol, Dilutes Thick Fats

This same garlic activator, diallyldisulfide, has the power to cleanse deposits from your bloodstream, thereby lowering your serum cholesterol levels. This garlic "scrubber" synthesizes (breaks down) wastes and fatty deposits in your liver. Garlic brings about a reduction of toxic wastes that otherwise threaten to clutter your bloodstream and heart. Garlic also reduces deposition levels of triglycerides (other forms of fatty wastes) in your bloodstream. You are then protected from toxic overload that could predispose you to heart trouble. Garlic is the pungent protector of your heart—and life.

How to Use Heart-Washing Garlic

Chew several cloves of garlic a day. Or chop a garlic bulb very finely and add to a salad, stew, casserole soup, or main dish. You may also press out garlic juice (a special garlic press is available at health stores and housewares outlets) and mix with a glass of vegetable juice. Drink one glass daily. The garlic compounds work vigorously and speedily to bring down your toxic levels and protect your heart from corrosive attack.

Garlic at Night = Heart Health at Daybreak

About two hours before going to sleep, consume four or five cloves of garlic. (Chew parsley or cloves to neutralize the anti-social odor.) Or else, chop the garlic finely and add to a raw lettuce and tomato salad. Eat before retiring for the night.

While you sleep the detoxifying elements in the garlic work with super-energy because competing digestive processes are now at rest. Consequently, undiluted energy can be mustered full force for the heart-scrubbing reaction. During your eight hours of sleep, the garlic compounds are washing away toxic wastes. Upon awakening, you'll have a cleaner heart. More youthful vitality, too.

THE SUPER-CLEANSING FOOD THAT REJUVENATES YOUR HEART POWER

An amazingly powerful super-cleansing food is able to dilute and discharge obstructive sludge deposits from your cardiovascular system and give your heart twice as much youthful power. This food works immediately.

Meet This Super-Cleanser

The name is *lecithin* (pronounced less-i-thin), it is a bland, water-soluble granular powder made from defatted soybeans or sunflower seeds. Cardiologists call it a *phosphatide;* that is, a waste-cleansing substance that detoxifies your cells, tissues, organs.

Lecithin's secret is in its *phospholipid* (fat-melting, waste-washing) power. This unique power enables this wonder food to melt away stubborn fats and wastes and detoxify your cardiovascular system.

The amazing power of lecithin is in its function as an emulsifier. It keeps fats and wastes broken up into microscopic particles so they can be detoxified and removed through arterial walls. *Protective Factor:* Lecithin searches out, then breaks down plaques (fibrous clumps that stick to your cardiovascular system) so they can be washed right out of your body. Lecithin is your super-cleansing heart food.

Choline, Cleansing, Clumping

Lester Morrison, M.D., of the Loma Linda (California) University School of Medicine, has found that lecithin works wonders in preventing and even reversing heart distress. The detoxification power is in its choline content.

"Choline causes a marked improvement of the blood flow properties in people with poor circulation. One hindrance to normal circulation is the tendency of platelets (blood cells) to clump together and form clots. Called 'platelet aggregability,' it is a risk. Choline (in lecithin) helps to keep the platelets from clumping together. This illustrates the point that choline does not actually 'thin' the blood. That is, it doesn't *remove* any of the platelets (which is good because they're necessary); it helps to keep them from clumping together."

Dr. Morrison cheers lecithin as an amazing food that is needed to help keep your heart cleansed and waste-free! [17]

STIMULATE INNER CLEANSING IN MINUTES

Lecithin—Your Heart Cleanser

Your heart requires a special enzyme called *lecithin cholesterol acyltransferase* (LCAT) in order to protect against excessive accumulation of waste on arterial walls. LCAT detoxifies and scrubs by keeping wastes from gluing together, by emulsifying them so they can be washed out.

Special Need: In order for your body to make this self-scrubbing LCAT, it requires lecithin. With this super-food, a unique detoxification takes place. Lecithin prompts body substances to work as intracellular "bouncers" that displace and discharge undesirable wastes and fatty plaques. It becomes your heart-saver . . . and life-saver, too.

Easy Way to Feed Yourself Cleansing Lecithin

Available at health stores, choose lecithin granules. They offer you a high potency of phosphatides and phosphatidylcholine—the powerhouses behind the scrubbing action.

How to Use: At breakfast, add four tablespoons of the granules to your breakfast cereal. At noontime, sprinkle two tablespoons over your fruit or vegetable salad. At dinnertime, add four tablespoons to your salad, main dish, or both.

Swift Reaction: Within moments after swallowing, the scrubbing substances in lecithin begin to cleanse your arteries and heart. You'll feel better almost at once. They continue scrubbing *overnight*. You will wake up feeling younger, your heart and body detoxified thanks to lecithin.

You Can See the Scrubbing Power of Lecithin

When you roast a fatty cut of meat, let the juices collect in a pan and cool off. Note that the fatty globules rise to the top. Now sprinkle one tablespoon of lecithin on top of the fat. Wait for 20 to 30 minutes. You'll discover that the fat has *disappeared*! The juices are there, but where is the fat? The lecithin has emulsified the fat, broken down the wastes, prepared them for swift disposal.

The same cleansing action occurs when you use lecithin in your meals. It will break up plaques and prompt a scrubbing power to give you a cleaner cardiovascular system almost overnight.

Simple Detoxification Program

Plan to use eight to ten tablespoons of lecithin granules daily. Gradually, as you experience improved heart health, better oxygenation, and better energy, your intake can be lowered to four tablespoons daily. Simple and tasty, these granules provide a heart-scrubbing and artery-cleansing detoxification that cannot be equalled. Lecithin may well be the super-food to give you a clean heart . . . and a healthier lifestyle.

CASE HISTORY—Cleans "Choked" Heart Within 48 Hours

Shortness of breath, palpitations of the heart, and chest tightening made Nora DeL. fearful she was developing cardiac difficulties. A physiologist told the housewife she had accumulations of waste plaques that needed to be eliminated immediately. He told her to restrict waste-forming foods from animal sources and boost the waste-washing foods from plant sources. Furthermore, she was told to take 10 tablespoons of lecithin granules daily. Nora DeL. wanted—and needed—swift action. She immediately took the granules, about 3 tablespoons with each meal. Some 48 hours later, she returned to her physiologist. It was amazing. The sludge had been washed right out of her body. She could breathe deeply, enjoyed a smoothly functioning heart. She had a "comfortable" chest, free of fearsome pains. All this took place within 48 hours. Nora DeL. has lecithin to thank for detoxifying her "choked" heart and giving her a healthier life ahead.

REVERSE HEART DISEASE . . . NATURALLY!

By following a set of detoxification programs to improve your lifestyle, you can correct your cholesterol, avoid heart disease, reverse (yes, reverse!) heart trouble, cut down, and eliminate medication and even bypass surgery!

This set of detoxification programs has worked for hundreds—even thousands—of people, says Dean Ornish, M.D., assistant clinical professor at the University of California, San Francisco and at the Pacific Presbyterian Medical Center.

Dr. Ornish's research suggests that diet and behavior changes can significantly reverse coronary blockages in only one year. He presents many of his patients as evidence that the programs can work! Many of them had high degrees of atherosclerosis or else had survived one or more heart attacks; others either refused or who for medical reasons could not undergo coronary bypass surgery to open their blockages. He developed his detoxification program that has saved countless lives.

The Fat Limit

Animal fats are taboo! The program emphasizes a supervised strict vegetarian diet deriving fewer than 10 percent of its calories from fat. Dr. Ornish tells of many of his patients who had reversal of coronary blockages. "As a result, people began to feel better very quickly." Another astonishing result: The more severe the heart disease, the more dramatic the detoxification on this program. But the focus is on the 10 percent of calories from fat! Yes, fat is the villain and must be rigidly controlled!

Before You Begin

"I say, just try it for one week," says Dr. Ornish. If you have angina and follow the program carefully, "after one week the pain will probably diminish. Even if you don't have heart disease at all, you'll feel noticeably better and have more energy after a week." But check with your health practitioner at the start. In either situation, a one-week test run will make you feel better.

Here is Dr. Dean Ornish's heart-smart program:

1. *Restrict Meats, High Fats.* Eliminate meat, poultry, fish, cheese. Go easy on high-fat vegetable products such as nuts, seeds, and vegetable oils. Avoid caffeinated coffee and teas. Caffeine may trigger irregular heartbeats in some people and lead to stress by giving you the jitters.
2. *Eat All You Want of These Foods:* Whole grains and whole grain products such as bread, cereal, brown rice, pasta, tortillas; fresh or dried fruits; greens and vegetables; beans; sprouts; egg whites. Many processed and convenience foods are acceptable if they have no added oil or egg yolks and only a minimum of sugar and salt. Acceptable are seasonings like herbs, mustard, salsa, and ketchup.
3. *What About Salt?* The program does not restrict salt. But if you are salt-sensitive, if your blood pressure responds to sodium levels, be cautious about avoiding it.

4. *Exercise In Moderation.* Dr. Ornish says, "The equivalent of walking a half-hour to one hour a day causes the greatest reduction in mortality. And beyond that you really don't get much more benefit, but the risks may go up substantially, especially for someone with severe heart disease." Plan to walk 20 to 30 minutes at the start at a pace that is comfortable. Work up to brisk walks of 30 to 60 minutes daily. Again, if you have heart problems, check with your doctor before you start any exercise program, even for a few days.

5. *Yoga Is Cleansing.* On a daily basis, try yoga stretches, which are best learned in a class with an instructor. Also available are tapes, audio and video. The rule is NOT to do anything that feels uncomfortable. When you stretch and a feeling of comfort makes you sigh, you're doing it properly.

6. *Cleansing Breaths.* Dr. Ornish advises this detoxification method which uses breathing. *First:* Sit up straight in a chair. Keep spine erect, shoulders back. Head is centered. Exhale completely. Breathe in, feel your abdomen expand. Exhale completely. Feel your abdomen pulling toward your spine. Repeat several times until this expansion-contraction detoxification occurs naturally. Then bring breathing back to normal and relax. *Second:* Exhale completely. Keep on inhaling fully, with your abdomen expanding, and your ribcage muscles expanding outward. When you exhale, feel your ribcage muscles contract, while your abdomen pulls in. This is a two-part detoxification oxygen program that combines movements of your abdomen and ribs. Repeat five times. Bring breathing back to normal and relax. *Third:* Place your hands on your collarbones. Exhale completely. Inhale. Feel your abdomen expand, your rib cage open, your collarbone rise. As you exhale, your collarbones rise slightly, your ribcage contracts and your abdomen pulls back. (After you have mastered this technique, you no longer have to hold your collarbones but can put your hands on your lap.) That's all there is to it. Dr. Ornish suggests breathing regularly, especially when stressed. It promotes a detoxification benefit to counteract tension. Plan at least 20 minutes a day for this three-step yoga remedy.

7. *Meditation Is Soothing.* Sit comfortably in a quiet place with your spine straight. If you do not want a chair, try the floor but put a firm cushion under your hips for comfort. Focus on your breathing. Rhythmically breathe in and out. Then conjure a word or sound and repeat it silently *as you breathe out.* Any word will do. Try "health," "detoxification," "cleansing," "love," "peace."—or whatever makes you feel good. Boost the detoxification by visualizing a relaxing scene. Do NOT

let your thoughts wander. Immerse yourself in this meditation-detoxification remedy. *Tip:* Meditate every day at the same time and place. You should wait several hours after eating. Aim to meditate for at least one 20-minute sitting each day.

8. *Group Support Is a Booster.* Try to get involved with others. Improve the lines of communications with family and friends. Isolated? Lonely? Become involved with other people. Doing so will help your heart. Dr. Ornish points out, "Can you do it on your own? Yes. Is it easier if you have a group? Yes. But it doesn't have to be a group of heart patients. It can be any kind of group. The idea is to be in a group that feels safe enough for you to show who you really are under the masks and defenses, and rather than feeling rejected, feel supported. That in itself is healing."[18]

FISH OILS DETOXIFY YOUR HEART

Among some populations, the increased intake of fish oils appears to protect against cardiovascular disease. Omega-3 fatty acids are cleansers found in fish oils that are important in protecting against coagulation. The same Omega-3 fatty acids are effective in lowering lipid (fat) levels. Fish oil has two detoxification benefits: (1) It lowers triclyceride-cholesterol levels; and (2) it minimizes formation of sludge-caused blood clots. *Important:* you cannot take fish oil and go on eating fatty foods. The cleansing comes from *substituting* fish for the foods that are fatty.

- It is the fish itself, not any oils it may be packed in, that is of primary benefit. Choose canned fish (sardines, mackerel, salmon, etc.) packed in water or tomato sauce.

- Fresh fish is beneficial, of course. Select from these Omega-3 fatty acid-containing fish: tuna, mackerel, salmon, bluefish, sardines, mullet, rainbow trout, lake trout, herring, sablefish, shad, butterfish, pompano. *Benefit:* These fish contain ample amounts of two fatty acids, eicosapentaenoic (EPA) and docosahexaenoic (DHA) that are vigorous detoxifying agents to help keep your arteries clean and reduce risk of heart trouble.

Fish will reduce both the numbers and stickiness of clot-forming blood platelets. The EPA and DHA in the Omega-3 fatty acids reduce the formation of artery-clogging fatty plaques on the walls of blood vessels and counter arterial spasms that interfere with blood flow and raise blood pressure.

What About Pollutants in Waters?

Vary the fish you eat. Some may be contaminated with certain pollutants. Fresh-water fish are especially likely to be contaminated by the toxic substances dumped into lakes, streams, and rivers. Ocean fish generally have less of a pollution problem, but the larger predator fish (tuna, swordfish) will accumulate chemical pollutants. NEVER eat raw fish since some contain infectious parasites.

AN ONION A DAY KEEPS YOUR HEART DOCTOR AWAY

Shed no tears over the pungent onion. Instead, be grateful for this aromatic vegetable—it has the power of cleansing your heart with such thoroughness, it can help keep your heart doctor away.

Melts Fats, Cleans and Breaks Down Sludge

The onion contains enzymes able to melt away accumulated fats and scrub them right out of your cardiovascular system. These onion enzymes shrink down plaque-like fibrin which might otherwise induce a dangerous blood clot.

The onion contains a hormone-like substance, *prostaglandin*. This substance cleans sludge from your blood, bringing fresh oxygen and nutrition to your heart.

Onion compounds reduce platelet aggregation sludge by breaking down a dangerous waste called *thromboxane*. By suppressing the multiplication of this waste, onion enzymes stimulate internal cleansing to protect your heart. Onion enzymes break up the "dams" of small blood clots (thrombi), which would otherwise gather and cause heart trouble. Just eating onions daily can help your body maintain this self-cleansing heart action.

Look (If You Can) at the Waste-Washing Power of Onions

Slice up a fresh onion. In seconds, your eyes start to water. The aroma of this all-powerful cleanser is so pungent that without even touching your eyes, it stimulates your lacrimal glands to release tears that wash away debris from your sight organs. The same reaction occurs when you *eat* onions. Their enzymes stimulate a melting down and washing out of accumulated debris. Like internal sprinklers, the enzymes wash and cleanse your cardiovascular system and eliminate the sludge. Eat onions regularly for this internal heart-washing detoxification to take place.

Onion Eating Plan

Use any seasonal raw onions as part of a vegetable salad daily. Or, use onions in cooking. Their detoxification powers are effective when cooked, too. Are you bothered because they make you weep on the outside when you would prefer this weeping (cleansing) inside? Then refrigerate the onion before slicing to inhibit its tear-inducing powers. Or, cut the onion under water for the same benefit. Eat one to two onions daily as part of your vegetable plan. Your heart will be all the cleaner.

All-Natural Heart Cleansing Tonic

Add two tablespoons of lecithin granules and one sliced or diced onion to a tall glass of fresh vegetable juice. Blenderize. Drink one glass daily.

CASE HISTORY—Revives Heart, Boosts Health in Three Days

Chest weakness and difficulty in breathing made Phyllis MacB. fearful that her heart was acting up on her. Since three family members had cardiac difficulties, she worried she would be next. Her internist said the problem stemmed from her clogged arterioles and heart valves. He put Phyllis MacB. on a detoxification program that emphasized more plant foods. He also prescribed the "All-Natural Heart Cleansing Tonic," to be taken twice daily. Within one day, Phyllis MacB. could breathe better. Her chest weakness was overcome. She had more youthful energy. At the end of three days, she was examined again. Her internist happily told her she had been so detoxified, she had excellent heart health. She resumed her regular activities with a new lease on life.

How Tonic Stimulates Heart Cleansing

The vitamin-mineral-enzyme combination of the lecithin and the onion as well as the juices invigorate the fat-fighting reaction in your body. This tonic uses lecithin to wash out fat and onion prostaglandin to accelerate heart cleansing. Within a short time after swallowing, this double-cleansing action is experienced. It works, often overnight, to give you a super-clean heart the next morning. And it's a refreshingly tasty tonic, too!

Detoxify Your Heart, Unclog Your Bloodstream While You Sleep

With the use of these detoxification programs, you can cleanse your heart and bloodstream while you sleep. Give your body the cleansing materials required for this lifesaving reaction. Your heart will then last nine lives . . . and then some.

───────────── *HIGHLIGHTS* ─────────────

1. *A clean heart is a healthy heart. Avoid sludge-forming "no-no" foods to add years to your heart.*

2. *Limit or eliminate waste-forming foods and boost intake of waste-cleaning foods. They wash your heart while you sleep.*

3. *Henry O'H. used the beneficial cleaning foods to go from "choked breath" to "vitality" within 48 hours.*

4. *Potassium is a powerful heart cleanser. Eat an assortment of foods containing potassium to keep cells free of toxins and protect against stroke.*

5. *Enjoy the Heart-Cleansing Potassium Broth. Delicious—lifesaving!*

6. *Garlic is a dynamic heart-cleanser. Take it at night and have a healthier heart by morning.*

7. *Lecithin is a super detoxifier for your heart and total body.*

8. *Nora DeL. cleaned her "choked" heart within 48 hours with a dietary change and the use of lecithin.*

9. *Reverse heart disease naturally (and build immunity to cardiovascular problems) with a doctor's eight-step detoxification program.*

10. *Seafood contains certain fatty acids that can detoxify your heart and unplug your arteries.*

11. *The humble onion is a powerful heart cleanser. In combination with lecithin, in an "All-Natural Heart Cleansing Tonic," it restored cardiovascular health to Phyllis MacB. within three days.*

Chapter 9

MIRACLE POWER FOODS FOR DYNAMIC CIRCULATION

Wash out toxic accumulations from your body and you rejuvenate your sluggish circulation. A toxin can be as insidious as the invisible pollutants seeping from the dust of your old building or as seemingly harmless as a cool (but poison-laden) breeze coming through your open window. Bacteria and viruses also add to the threat of body pollution. You can minimize these threats with a stepped-up program to detoxify your system and cleanse your organs.

When free-flowing, refreshingly oxygenated blood travels throughout your body, your trillions of cells and tissues become free of blockages. You are rewarded with the look and feel of youthful health. You can experience this "reborn" feeling with miracle power foods that give you a dynamic circulation.

HOW FOODS BOOST YOUTHFUL CIRCULATION

Certain everyday foods and nutrients have built-in natural substances that wash away the toxic wastes that threaten to impede your circulatory system. These foods can gently and thoroughly scrub out and dislodge the glue-like encumbrances that interfere with free-flowing circulation. Once these foods have cleansed your inner pathways, you can enjoy health-boosting regeneration through youthful (and youth-building) circulation.

Speedy Detoxification = Dynamic Circulation

These miracle power foods aim directly at removing blockages from the clogged pathways which might otherwise block the movement of important nutrients. These same foods actually widen the arteries and veins of your circulatory system to promote a better exchange of waste products and oxygen to give you a cleaner and more youthful metabolism. These miracle foods cleanse the toxin-clogged pathways to speed up the vigorous transport of wastes for elimination.

Swift Cleansing, Immediate Total Alertness

The enzymatic catalysts in these miracle foods create swift inner cleansing. They work to regenerate damaged and broken capillaries almost from the start. They cleanse the smallest components of your vascular system. Inner cleansing allows for an exchange of oxygen for wastes through the semipermeable walls of your capillaries. Basically, a constant breakdown of capillaries will reduce their filtering efficiency. These walls become toxin-laden, creating blockages which can weaken the cleansing process that is vital for maintaining youthful health. Therefore, you need to take in nutrients that will (1) dispatch and disperse accumulated wastes, and (2) repair your capillaries so they become strong and can function as efficient filters. With these miracle foods, you experience inner cleansing and repair and immediate youthful alertness.

ONE-DAY GRAPE JUICE FAST = FOREVER YOUNG CIRCULATION

Mark your calendar. Every ten days, schedule a grape juice fast for just one day. Take no foods and no other liquids except water. Throughout this entire day, drink unsweetened grape juice.

Cleanses, Rejuvenates, Exhilarates Circulation

The rich concentration of enzymes, combined with the high vitamin C content, work swiftly to cleanse accumulated wastes from the nooks and crannies of your circulatory network. The grape juice enzymes stimulate gastric secretions and motility to speed up the inner cleansing. The enzymes and the vitamin C also stimulate an antibacterial action that prompts a natural colonic cleansing which is then better able to discharge the waste products that might otherwise cause circulatory blockages.

Without the digestive competition of other foods and beverages, your enzymatic system is able to make full use of the grape juice nutrients to bring about this cleansing reaction. You will feel rejuvenated as you enjoy a more exhilarating and sparkling clean circulation.

One Day Creates Lifetime Wonder

This one day (scheduled every ten days on your calendar) can so supercharge your gastroenteric functions that you experience the lifetime wonder of youthful circulation. Plan to follow this naturally sweet and speedily cleansing grape juice fast program regularly, and you will be rewarded with a feeling of total youth.

CASE HISTORY—**Firms Skin, Enjoys Regularity, Doubles Energy**

Bookkeeper Frank E.P. complained of feeling "clogged up." He had sagging skin, discomforting irregularity, and a low energy level. As the days wore on, he became wearier and wearier. At times, the long debit-credit columns seemed to grow blurry before his bloodshot eyes. Frank E.P.'s work productivity declined. Confiding his problems in his supervisor, he was told to visit the company physiologist. Tests showed his circulation was "choked" with blockages of wastes from end products of improperly metabolized foods. Environmental pollution from office machines, chemical fumes from industries in the area, and toxic substances inhaled with each breath compounded the problem. Frank E.P. was told to go on a simple one-day grape juice fast every other week. He followed this simple program. He was amazed when he felt energy rebounding. His skin became firm and smooth. He achieved regularity. He not only went through his balance sheet preparation speedily, he could work overtime with twice as much energy. He thanks this circulation-cleansing one-day grape juice fast as the key to his refreshing feeling of "total rejuvenation."

"EARLY MORNING CIRCULATION BOOSTER"

The rate of circulation while you sleep varies from the rate during the daytime. There are days when accumulation of wastes become blockages, making it difficult for you to get started in the morning. You know how it feels. You can hardly get out of bed! You need to wash away these accumulations. You can boost your circulation with the use of four everyday miracle power foods in a dynamic combination.

How to Prepare Booster

> 1 cup fresh orange juice
> 1 teaspoon brewer's yeast (from health store)
> 2 teaspoons fortified non-fat powdered milk
> 1 egg white (give yolk to family pet)

Blenderize all ingredients for 30 seconds. Then sip slowly before you have breakfast. (Works best on an empty stomach in the morning.)

Cleansing-Energizing Benefits

The invigorating vitamin C of the orange juice combines with the powerful B-complex and amino acids of the yeast. They boost the rich protein concentration of the milk and egg white to create an almost instant cell-scrubbing reaction. These same dynamic ingredients surge through your circulatory system, sweeping away wastes, waking up your sluggish metabolism, filling your bloodstream with throbbing vitality. Within 30 minutes after you finish this Early Morning Circulation Booster, you will experience a revival of dynamic energy. This is a reward for having cleansed your circulatory system upon awakening.

CASE HISTORY—**Booster Gives Her Unlimited "Get Up and Go"**

Diane O'J. felt mounting responsibilities of home, local social affairs, and a part-time job. These tasks took such a toll, she wanted to sleep all the time. She would wake up tired and remain fatigued as she forced herself through daily chores—family and job. She walked with a stooped gait and was slow with her reflexes. Her memory was vague. She was in her forties but felt twice as old! A sympathetic co-worker suggested she use the easily prepared "Early Morning Circulation Booster" that had been prescribed by a clinical nutritionist for her own sluggishness. Diane O'J. tried it, desperate to get out of her slump. Within two days, she was completely refreshed. She enjoyed her many activities. She walked with a youthful bounce, had sharper reflexes, a much better memory. The tasty booster had reversed her aging process and rewarded her with unlimited "get up and go." Life was so joyful!

LIMIT (OR ELIMINATE) THESE CIRCULATION-BLOCKING FOODS

To help keep your circulation unblocked, restrict these "glue-like" foods that dump heavy burdens of waste and toxic deposits at vital checkpoints throughout your system:

- Whole milk, chocolate milk, malts, shakes, heavy cream.
- Luncheon meats, sausages, frankfurters, heavily marbled meats, poultry with skin, pan- or deep-fried meats, commercially prepared meats, poultry with breading, gravies.
- Frozen or canned vegetables that are in butter or cream sauce, that are deep fried, or that contain added salt and chemicals.
- Bread products (bread, biscuits, muffins, pancakes, waffles, doughnuts) made with cream, whole milk, animal fats, chemicals.
- Coconut oil, cocoa butter, palm oil, hydrogenated or "hardened" vegetable shortening, meat drippings, suet, or lard.

- Commercially prepared gravies or sauces. If homemade, avoid those containing large proportions of animal fats, salt, harsh seasonings.
- Ice cream, whipped cream, ice milk, or frozen desserts containing above named animal or "hard" fats.
- Chocolate, fudge, caramels, custard and pudding made with whole milk, commercial cakes, pies, cookies, and mixes of unknown ingredients.
- Commercially fried foods such as potato chips and other snacks which have been dunked in toxemia-causing fats.

Why Are These Harmful Foods?

These foods are concentrated sources of hard fats and additives that leave thick deposits of sludge throughout your circulatory system. Continual intake of these waste-forming foods causes a "pile-up" of blockage-forming debris. Your circulation is at risk of being narrowed down or choked off completely. This takes its toll in your cellular rejuvenation process. Do not assault your circulatory system with food pollution. Limit, or better yet, *eliminate* these "no-no" foods. You will then limit waste accumulation and give your circulation the free-flowing power it needs to give you a feeling of revived youth.

POWER HERBS TO SUPERCHARGE YOUR CIRCULATION

Various herbs have the power to revive your sluggish circulation, warm your hands and feet, and make you feel glad all over. These herbs are available at many health stores as well as from herbal pharmacists.

Cold Limbs. To warm hands and feet, massage gently with warmed macerated oil of honeysuckle flowers. *Benefit:* Stimulates an increased blood flow to your skin surface.

Foot Bath. Warm up your cold feet by soaking them in two quarts warm water to which you add an infusion of one tablespoon freshly ground mustard seed. Only 30 minutes and circulation zooms to give you warm feet. *Benefit:* Herb cleanses while it stimulates.

Herb Tonic. Drink rose hips tea, or field horsetail tea, with a bit of honey and lemon juice. *Benefit:* Strengthens and cleanses small capillaries to improve flow of oxygen-bearing nutrients.

NUTRIENTS THAT STRENGTHEN YOUR BREATHING POWER

Importance of Healthy Lungs

Robert H. Garrison, Jr., registered pharmacist of San Diego, California and Elizabeth Somer, registered dietitian, authors of *The Nutrition Desk Reference* call for inner cleansing of the lungs as a gateway to improved health.

"The lungs are exposed to numerous environmental substances that can cause infection and damage, including molds, bacteria, viruses, pollen, air pollutants, and tobacco smoke. Tobacco use and secondhand smoke are the greatest contributors to bronchitis, emphysema, and lung cancer.

"The barriers to infection and tissue damage include enzymes that destroy foreign substances, a strong epithelial lining that forms a physical barrier to contaminants, a mucus coating that covers the epithelial lining and further discourages invasion, and a layer of minute hairlike structures called cilia on the lining of the respiratory tract. Cilia brush away debris that has been inhaled. The immune system and antioxidant system also help protect the lungs from damage."

The registered pharmacist and dietitian team point out, "Good nutrition helps maintain healthy lung tissue by strengthening the immune system and increasing the body's resistance to infection and disease, maintaining a healthy epithelial lining, and deactivating free radicals and other highly reactive compounds that might damage lung tissue and possibly cause cancer."

Which nutrients and foods? The most powerful inner cleansers they recommend include:

1. *Vitamin A and its precursor beta-carotene.* This nutrient is essential for normal development and maintenance of epithelial tissue and mucous membranes, including the lining of the lungs, bronchi, and other respiratory tissues. "These epithelial tissues form a barrier to bacteria and other pathogens and help in the prevention of infection and disease. Vitamin A and beta-carotene also contribute to a well-functioning immune system and thus provide a secondary influence on resistance to lung disorders. Beta-carotene is particularly effective in preventing cancers of the lung," say the experts. *Food Sources:* Vitamin A is found in liver, eggs, cheese, fortified dairy and margarine products (but these are also high in fat). Beta-carotene is found in yellow, orange, and dark green vegetables and fruits (carrots, broccoli, sweet potato, cantaloupe).

2. *Vitamin E.* The nutrition experts tell us, "The antioxidant effects of vitamin E help protect cell membranes in the lungs from damage caused by air pollutants and tobacco smoke. People with lung cancer have lower levels of vitamin E in their tissue than do healthy people." *Food Sources:* Vegetable oils, wheat germ, whole grain breads and cereals, leafy green vegetables.

3. *Minerals.* They explain, "Inadequate intake of copper during the early stages of development might be linked to later occurrence of lung damage similar to emphysema. Iron, manganese, and zinc are essential trace minerals for the maintenance of a strong immune system and help protect all tissues, such as those in the lungs, that form a barrier to the environment. Selenium deficiency is associated with increased risk for developing lung cancer. Blood levels of this mineral (selenium) are low in people who subsequently develop cancer." *Food Sources:* Fresh fruits and vegetables, whole grains, brewer's yeast. Supplements are available to be used in conjunction with advice from your health practitioner.[19]

THE CLOT-CLEANSING VITAMIN THAT MAY SAVE YOUR LIFE

When excess wastes are allowed to accumulate, they force the blood to form clots. These waste-filled clots become dangerous blockades in the bloodstream; that is, they block the free flow of circulating blood. Furthermore, these same wastes are glue-like in that they force blood cells (called platelets) to stick together to become dangerous clots.

Glue-Filled Platelets Are Life Risk

If allowed to accumulate, these platelets do more than glue themselves together as a clot. They release granules containing a dangerous waste called lactic acid. This inner pollutant is a highly concentrated grain-like set of particles within the platelets. Once lactic acid breaks loose, it spreads to glue other platelets together. DANGER: They form clumps which block blood flow out of the vessel which leads to a possible stroke. So you can see the danger to your life if you have an excess of these glue-filled platelets.

Vitamin B₆ Is Super Cell Cleanser

This member of the B-complex family (also called pyridoxine) blocks the action of lactic acid. It cleanses the pollution-filled cells, and it controls the aggregation of the glue-like platelets. It dilutes lactic acid, stimulates its washing out of your body, and protects against a life-threatening clot. It has super cell cleansing power.

The higher the pyridoxine levels, the greater your protection against cellular pollution and the clot-causing lactic acid Vitamin B_6 (pyrodoxine) cleanses your cells and gives you a more vigorous and youthful circulation.

Food Sources of Cell-Cleansing Vitamin B_6

Include these foods in your menu for each day: whole grain breads and cereals, fish, poultry, bananas, nuts, potatoes, wheat germ, brewer's yeast. Supplements are available at health stores.

Boost your blood levels of vitamin B_6 and you boost your cell cleansing powers. You will protect yourself against the threat of a blood clot choking away your breath of life

CASE HISTORY—Breathes Better, Looks Younger, Feels Revived in Eight Days

Shortness of breath and chronic fatigue sent Ned DiN. to his respiratory specialist. Tests showed he had a dangerously high level of glue-like platelet clumps. Their released particles caused circulatory blockages, the reason for his illness. The specialist put him on a high vitamin B_6 program. Each day he was to eat an assortment of the foods containing this cell cleanser. Ned DiN. started to breathe better almost at once. Fatigue was gone. He enjoyed unusual vitality. He glowed with youthful health. Within eight days, he felt "eighty years younger," as he quipped, thanks to the detoxification power of this amazing vitamin.

"Triple Circulation Pick-Up Elixir"

You can "pick up" your circulation when you super-clean your cells with this tasty and invigorating elixir.

> 1 cup grapefruit juice
> 3 teaspoons fortified
>   non-fat powdered milk
> 1 teaspoon wheat germ
> 1 teaspoon bran
> 1/2 banana
> 1 egg white (give yolk to family pet)

Blenderize all ingredients for 30 seconds. Drink one glass at noontime each day.

Inner Cleansing Benefits

The rich concentration of vitamin C plus pectin (a powerful cell cleanser and rebuilder) of the grapefruit juice activates the protein of the milk to join with the pyridoxine of the grains. With the minerals in the banana and the complete protein of the egg white, they actually scour your circulatory system. This Elixir propels wastes right out of your system. The rich concentration of natural fruit sugars works to energize your circulatory system. Soon you feel a flow of vitality that makes you act with youthful vigor. Clean circulation gives you this picked-up feeling.

The Triple Circulation Pick-Up Elixir does, in effect, triple the vigor of your circulation to give you a head-to-toe lively, healthy feeling.

CASE HISTORY—Instant Vigor with Elixir

Stooped shoulders, a hangdog expression, and chronic fatigue so upset Olga B.Y., that she became a recluse. She could hardly keep up with others. In her isolation she listened to the radio, which was the only company she had. She heard an interviewed nutritionist tell of the "Triple Circulation Pick-Up Elixir," and how it initiated inner cleansing. It boosted energy powers of the circulatory system. Olga B.Y. decided to give it a try. She prepared it right away. Almost from the start, she felt a restoration of energy. Her face brightened up. She could walk erectly, with more vigor. She would drink the elixir twice daily. Within three days, she was so full of life, she went disco dancing . . . with folks much younger than herself. When she won a prize, she said her secret was "triple circulation" power. The elixir had, indeed, picked her up and made her look and act alive again with renewed vigor

Beware of Poor Circulation

People with circulation problems often develop phlebitis, blood clots in the veins of their legs or arms. The clots cause limbs to swell, as stagnant blood leaks through vessel walls into surrounding tissue. Unblock those waste deposits. Set your circulation free. Let oxygen transport energy-boosting nutrients and cell-repairing elements throughout your body. With the use of miracle power foods, you will experience dynamic circulation rejuvenation. Enjoy this restoration of total youth.

———————————— *HIGHLIGHTS* ————————————

1. Cleanse circulation blockages with an occasional one-day grape juice fast. It rejuvenated Frank E.P. and gave him the breath of life.

2. *Wake up your sluggish responses with an "Early Morning Circulation Booster." It scrubs your cells, gives you powerful vigor. It gave fatigue-plagued Diane O'J. unlimited "get up and go."*

3. *Avoid those circulation-blocking foods as listed in this chapter. These "no-no" foods are to blame for inner body pollution.*

4. *Power herbs supercharge your circulation.*

5. *A set of nutrients found in everyday foods will strengthen your breathing powers and invigorate your circulation.*

6. *Ned DiN. used vitamin B_6 (pyridoxine) as a super cell cleanser and enjoyed restored and revived circulation with youthful vitality in only eight days.*

7. *Olga B.Y. overcame her premature aging and chronic tiredness with a tasty "Triple Circulation Pick-Up Elixir," within three days.*

Chapter 10

HOW TO "UNLOCK" AND "RELEASE" WASTES FOR FREEDOM FROM "AGING STIFFNESS"

An accumulation of wastes that cling stubbornly to the multicellular components of your joints can be the underlying cause of your complaints of muscle stiffness. These leftover byproducts of internal combustion back up and block the free passage of oxygen and circulating blood. These wastes interfere with nourishment of your joints and muscles. They choke your circulatory system at vital depots and create such blockages that you wince with pain if you have to reach for an object on a high shelf, or if you need to bend at the waist to look in a low shelf. This indicates your cellular system has become heavily laden with these waste byproducts.

Daily Usage Causes Toxic Waste Backup

As you perform your daily chores, whether mild or vigorous, you use your entire set of joints and muscles. To energize these segments, a biological reaction occurs. There is a transformation of adenosine triphosphate (ATP) into adenosine diphosphate (ADP). This gives you the energy needed to use your joints and muscles. In the meantime, this process also deposits a substance called *lactic acid,* which actually is a toxic waste. It exists only as part of the biological process of supplying energy; it is refuse left behind that needs to be eliminated. It is this lactic acid that often accumulates and creates toxic waste backup. In brief, lactic acid is a substance that forms in the cells as the end product of glucose metabolism in the absence of oxygen. During strenuous physical movement or exercise, pyruvic acid (a compound derived from carbohydrates) is reduced to lactic acid, which may accumulate in the muscles and cause cramps. Therefore, lactic acid is a byproduct of metabolism; it may accumulate and contribute to "aging stiffness" and muscular fatigue.

Overload of Lactic Acid Is Tiring, Hurtful

The accumulation of lactic acid in muscle and blood can interfere with the nerve stimulation of muscle, the contraction process, and energy production. Interference with these processes can lead to "aging stiffness." But lactic acid is not useless. It does serve as an energy source, as a means of disposing of dietary carbohydrate, and as a building block for blood glucose and liver glycogen. When you have an overload, when the entry of lactic acid into the blood is greater than the removal rate, you become tired and lethargic, and you feel pain.

WASH OUT LACTIC ACID FOR GREATER JOINT-MUSCLE FLEXIBILITY

To put more flexibility into your joints and muscles you need to stimulate an internal cleansing action that washes out excessive lactic acid. In particular, you need to oxygenate your system so the waste can (1) be largely eliminated, and (2) be transformed into glycogen, a prime energy source. It is oxygen that will perform this double-action body energizer. That is, rid your body of the excessive lactic acid and then create glycogen which gives you youthful flexibility in your joints and muscles.

THE FOOD THAT WASHES WASTES AND REJUVENATES JOINTS

Lecithin is a power food. It is an emulsifier, rich in two B vitamins, inositol and choline. It works like soap in your bloodstream to emulsify fats and wastes, reducing them to a form that can be readily washed out, instead of coagulating in your arteries. Made from defatted soybeans or sunflower seeds, it is available at most health stores. It works speedily to wash your cells and tissues so you have more youthful flexibility in a short time.

Contains Powerful Waste-Washer

A bland, water-soluble food, lecithin contains a little-known substance called *acetylcholine*. This is a powerful waste-washer that can rejuvenate your body and provide you with superior joint/muscle flexibility almost as soon as it is consumed. Lecithin releases acetylcholine, which then triggers off the conversion of ATP to ADP. During this instantaneous process, the lecithin-distributed acetylcholine sweeps up lactic acid wastes, dilutes this sludge, and uses the energy-packed ADP to wash it right out of your body. Within minutes after you have eaten lecithin, this waste-washing process takes place. You will experience more flexibility in your joints and muscles so very rapidly. Lecithin is a super-cleanser and super-energizer because of this biological reaction.

Cleanses Brain, Liver, Bloodstream

This food actually helps revitalize your brain. Lecithin acetylcholine washes wastes from nerve cells to give you more reflex strength and better thinking ability. It further works to metabolize accumulated fat from your liver and protects against buildup of wastes that may lead to degeneration of this vital organ. Lecithin acetylcholine also acts as a guard in washing away fat that might otherwise accumulate in your bloodstream to be deposited in your arteries. So you can readily appreciate the dynamic overall cleansing power of lecithin.

HOW TO USE LECITHIN FOR SPEEDY JOINT-MUSCLE ENERGY

To reverse the "aging" of your joints and muscles, use lecithin daily to wash away excessive lactic acid accumulations.

Easy Way to Enjoy Lecithin

Sprinkle several teaspoons of lecithin granules in soups, on your salads (fruit or vegetables), in baked goods, in juices. Add to your cereals, hot or cold. Stir into any dairy dish, such as yogurt. Take advantage of lecithin's emulsifying powers by adding the granules in gravies, sauces, dressings. Even small amounts of lecithin can improve the workability of the batter of any baking mixture, and boost the quality of the finished product. Yes, you can *eat and clean your body at the same time,* when lecithin is part of the recipe.

(Energy Drink)

"INSTANT POWER POTION"

To a glass of fresh citrus juice, add two tablespoons of lecithin granules, a teaspoon of honey, one-half teaspoon of brewer's yeast. Blenderize for 30 seconds. Drink slowly.

Speedy Energy

Within moments after swallowing, the vitamin C of the juice invigorates the acetylcholine of the lecithin to wash away the lactic acid wastes from your joints and muscles. This combination is further energized by the concentrated minerals in the honey and the stimulation from the B-complex vitamins in the brewer's yeast. The benefit is a vigorous internal scouring that occurs within minutes. In a short time, your cleansed joints and muscles will feel youthfully flexible. You will be able to move with the agility of a youngster. Such is the power of this dynamic food combination.

Triple Your Energy With Easy Program

To enjoy triple energy, plan to drink the Instant Power Potion three times a day. After breakfast, at noontime, then in the early evening. You will be scrubbing away excessive lactic acid throughout the day. You will also transform the waste substance, ATP, into the energy producing ADP. This cleansing-energizing process will give you three-fold vitality throughout the day. Your joints and muscles will be flexible so you can fulfill your daily chores with the vitality of a youngster.

CASE HISTORY—From "Too Tired" to "Too Active" in Three Days

No matter what George E. had to do, he was always "too tired." His wife complained that work piled up because he could not muster enough strength to do the most simple tasks. He complained of stiff joints. His muscles ached if he carried a small bundle. At work as a factory foreman he became neglectful and let errors creep by because his body was always so "tight" that he could not make the necessary corrections. A neuromuscular physician diagnosed his problem as "cement-like" sludge accumulating on his joints and muscles. An excess of lactic acid was responsible for his chronic muscular fatigue. He prescribed the Instant Power Potion, three times daily. George E. began at once. From the start, he felt his joints and muscles loosening up. Within two days, he could do a good day's work at the factory and many chores at home at night. By the end of the third day, his "too tired" feeling had vanished. His co-workers and wife chided him for being "too active." The washing away of constricting and choking wastes gave him youthful flexibility. Lecithin was the power food!

HOW TO VENTILATE YOUR JOINTS FOR MORE YOUTHFUL MOBILITY

Simple body motions or exercises that you perform during your daily routine can send a stream of waste-washing oxygen throughout your body. Your goal is to *minimize* lactic acid production and *maximize* lactic acid removal. This inner cleansing is prompted by the rate of oxygen intake and blood lactic acid concentration. Because of that, it can be seen that increasing capacity of the pathways of lactic acid removal depends to a large extent on full ventilation or oxygenation of your joints. The key word is *activity*. When you keep physically active, the lactic acid is dispelled, the sludge byproducts of adenosine triphosphate (ATP) are washed away. Your circulatory system becomes refreshed. *Suggestion:* Fit the following easy and fun-to-do exercises into your daily schedule and be rewarded with more youthful mobility.

1. A railing is required for use as a dance bar. Grab onto the bar and kick your legs out behind you alternating left and right. Now turn and lift your legs out to the side, first facing the front of the room, then the back. Only five minutes daily boosts the cleansing process to limber up your tight muscles.

2. When in a warm tub, lift your legs and stretch your toes. The comfortable heat of the bath will unlock sludge and prepare it for evaporation while your taut muscles become more flexible.

3. After your bath, sit on the tub's edge. Stretch both arms in all directions. When drying yourself, hold the towel up around the back of your neck; move your arms from side to side, twisting your body from left to right as you dry off. This movement will exhilarate your entire body. (Your mind, too. It's all connected!)

4. When sweeping the floor (not enjoyable, but it can be made beneficial), use the broom as a support. Stretch your right leg backwards. Then reverse and stretch your left leg backwards. Keep doing this as you sweep—it oxygenates your system, makes sweeping more of an inner cleansing exercise than of a chore.

5. Frequently throughout the day, rise up and down on your toes. The accelerated breathing will oxygenate your circulatory system and ventilate your joints and muscles to promote flexibility.

With daily use of these body movements, you will give your joints and muscles a form of daily scrubbing that will make you feel flexible all over.

GARLIC: DYNAMIC WASTE-WATCHER

Garlic contains an anti-oxidant ingredient that is more than a waste-watcher—it is a waste-washer, too. The dynamic anti-oxidant power means that it is able to swoop down on wastes, such as peroxides, toxins, and free radicals (bits and scraps from incomplete metabolism) and keep them from accumulating to excess.

Garlic acts as a watchman. With its mitogenetic radiation factor, it prevents wastes from remaining too long in your joint/muscle system. Garlic uproots these ache- and pain-causing wastes and prepares them for elimination. Garlic, therefore, functions as a guard to protect your body against waste overload.

Eat Garlic Daily

Two or three well-chewed garlic cloves daily makes these waste-watching functions available to keep your cells clean. This easy and tasty program helps you enjoy a more flexible range of movement in your joints and muscles.

CASE HISTORY—Garlic Frees Joints from Stiffness

Waitress Dolores LaF. was warned that her job was in jeopardy because she could hardly carry even moderately heavy trays of food to the restaurant customers. Wiping off a table made her wince with pain because of her limited joint range; tears involuntarily came down her face, hardly an appetizing sight to customers. Complaining to a produce deliveryman, he told her that he, too, suffered from joint stiffness to the point where he doubled up in pain. Then he heard of garlic as a long-time remedy for muscular problems. He ate several cloves daily. Within a short time, he regained full use of his arms and legs. Dolores LaF. decided to try it. She also ate parsley or sometimes a cinnamon stick, to protect against garlic's offensive scent. Within four days, she was able to carry heavy trays with the greatest of ease. She could wash and clean and do kitchen chores with full joint/muscle range. Garlic had cleaned away the sediment that caused the stiffness. She could even work overtime—with nary a complaint, thanks to pain-easing garlic!

HOW TO RUB AWAY BRUISES AND SPRAINS

To help stimulate sluggish circulation and "rub" away lactic acid and other waste overload, try any of these rubs. The herbs are available at most health stores or herbal pharmacies.

- *Small Bumps, Bruises.* Apply distilled witch hazel with sterile cotton balls to small bumps and bruises. This halts the swelling.
- *Scrapes, Bruises, Sprains.* Rub on comfrey oil or comfrey ointment for speedy relief. A poultice of comfrey leaves will reduce bruising and

speed healing of sprains. *Careful:* Do not use on deep wounds. Comfrey is a powerful tissue healer, and the surface skin may heal before the wound has healed deeper down.

- *Sprains, Inflammation.* Rub on a lotion of St.-John's-wort, especially helpful if you have either inflammation or pain of the skin. You may also use a lotion of arnica as a cleansing-healing rub.
- *Muscle-Joint Ache.* An ointment of calendula petals, agrimony, or elder leaves helps soothe and promote healing of hurtful muscles or joints.
- *Painful Swelling.* Rub in several drops of eucalyptus oil. Easy does it . . . the pain will subside over a period of time. Repeat frequently.

The Liniment Mystique

Topical rubs or liniments are available in health stores and pharmacies. Basically, a liniment is helpful because it increases skin warmth and helps to push out stagnating particles from your body parts to provide relief. Popular liniments are wintergreen and eucalyptus oil, among others.

When you rub a liniment on the aching part, the skin becomes aroused, causing surrounding blood vessels to dilate. Your skin soon feels warm and muscular pain seems to lessen in the area as pain receptors become depressed. Actually, they stimulate sluggish nerves, causing the nerve receptors to ease the hurt.

When liniment is combined with some activity at a slow pace, followed by light stretching, you are able to help set off the metabolic reaction to wash out accumulated hurt-causing wastes.

Apply a bit of liniment to your palms and gently rub the aching part, using very moderate pressure. Move across the grain and perpendicular to the length of the muscle, or in a circular fashion. About 30 minutes a day will help cleanse away the hurtful particles of waste that are lodged in your muscles.

THE R.I.C.E. REMEDY FOR INNER CLEANSING

Listen to your body. Several signs will indicate to you that you have excessive sludge: persistent pain, inability to move certain body parts, sprains, strains, tenderness, inflammation. To help wash out the accumulated waste products, try the R.I.C.E. remedy. No, it does not mean eating rice (although that is a healthy energy-producing grain), but it refers to a four-step program to cleanse away grating sandpaper-like particles that cause pain.

1. *Rest.* As soon as you feel pain, stop what you are doing. Do not continue to stress the injured part for at least one day. However, except in severe strains, sprains, or injuries, complete and prolonged rest is not necessary unless prescribed by your health specialist. In fact, complete rest may allow buildup of metabolite fragments which can often be the wrong course of action.

   Within a few days after injury, the tissues begin to repair themselves; but there are byproducts of the injury that should be cleansed away. Comfortable exercise will help remove these wastes. Even if there is some minor hurt, the gentle movement will help restore the muscle's ability to function properly, allowing you to return to your activities that much sooner.

2. *Ice.* Put ice on the injured area, as soon as possible after the hurt. Wrap the ice in a towel or plastic bag and apply it over a 30-minute period. However, move it every five minutes so as to avoid frostbite. This process can be continued several times.

   Ice is important for inner cleansing. It reduces pain and swelling by constricting blood and lymph vessels. By reducing blood that collects around the injured area, there is less inflammation and subsequently less time is required for recovery.

3. *Compression.* Compression also helps limit swelling, which, if left uncontrolled, could lengthen healing time. Wrap an elastic bandage around the injured part. Be sure not to wrap too tightly—this could cut off the blood supply. The bandage is too tight if you feel numbness in the area, cramping, additional pain, or swelling beyond the edge of the bandage. Leave the bandage on for 30 minutes, then remove it for 15 minutes to ease circulation. *Tip:* The bandage may be applied over the ice.

4. *Elevation.* Elevating an injured leg or arm to above heart level helps drain excess waste-clogged fluid from the injured area. Both compression and elevation help limit muscular internal bleeding, decreasing the amount of injury byproducts that need to be removed while the area is repairing itself. You may continue to elevate the injured leg or arm even while sleeping.

As soon as you feel comfortable and unless your health specialist says otherwise, start gentle range-of-motion exercises (within limits of discomfort) to rehabilitate the injured joints, muscles, or arteries. The sooner you use your muscles, the sooner you are able to return to your normal activity and the less likelihood there is of your muscles weakening. However, moderation is important. Pain means you are overdoing it.

HOW TO STEAM WASTES OUT OF YOUR ACHING JOINTS

Luxuriate in a bath filled with comfortably warm water. It should be warm enough so that you perspire. This prompts an outpouring of melted-down joint-muscle wastes that are released through the steam-opened pores. Only 30 minutes will help steam clean most of the blockage-forming wastes out of your body. You'll emerge from the tub with more flexible joints and resilient muscles. If you wish, add fragrant herbs to the bathwater for more comfort and healing. CAUTION: Folks with heart problems, vascular disorders, or diabetes should use heat and/or ice with caution and only with the consent of their health practitioner.

ARE YOUR MUSCLES NUTRITIONALLY DEFICIENT?

Muscles and joints require an adequate amount of nutrition in order to function with flexibility. An ache may be a sign of nutritional deficiency. Feed your muscles and joints the essential elements required for waste cleansing and you are spared discomfort.

Muscles require an "electrolyte soup" of water, vitamins, potassium, magnesium, calcium, pantothenic acid, and other substances. Deficiency of any of these nutrients, or an imbalance, can lead to waste overload and symptoms such as fatigue, cramps, stiffness, and joint aches.

Boost the inner cleansing of your muscles and joints with these nutrients:

- *Water*—washes out accumulated wastes and is vital for moisturizing and quenching the thirst of your cells and tissues in the process of inner cleansing.
- *Vitamin C*—builds and rebuilds cell walls and manufactures collagen needed to strengthen your entire tissue network.
- *Potassium*—valuable electrolyte that is involved with other minerals for proper contraction and relaxation of your muscular system.
- *Magnesium*—protects against irregular heartbeat, muscle spasms, twitching, trembling, easily injured bones.
- *Calcium*—participates with other nutrients to build a strong skeletal structure; also needed for calming the nervous system.
- *Pantothenic Acid*—muscle is an abundant tissue in your body and your muscles require an adequate amount of this nutrient. It is needed for formation of steroid hormones since sludge tends to bring on a situation of stress and you secrete excessive amounts of adrenal cor-

tical hormones. Have pantothenic acid available to meet these needs or more wastes will accumulate.

- *Zinc*—mineral needed for joint cleansing. When the membranes of the joints become inflamed, zinc levels may be depleted. This mineral participates in the cleansing away of wastes so the inflammation is eased.
- *Selenium*—a micromineral that helps build an important protective enzyme system, glutathione peroxidase. The mineral strengthens the joint/muscular system with this enzyme system and initiates a cleansing response at the same time.

A balance of all the nutrients is needed in order to cleanse away the "locked" wastes and wash them out of your system. You can have a more flexible body with inner cleansing.

Remove the "rust" from your joints and muscles with nutritional help, simple exercises, herbal programs, and steaming and you will enjoy freedom from "aging stiffness."

HIGHLIGHTS

1. *Wear and tear of joints and muscles will cause lactic acid waste backup that interferes with flexibility.*
2. *Lecithin helps wash wastes out of your system and restore youthful movement to your limbs.*
3. *George E. went from "too tired" to "too active" in three days with the help of the cleansing and tasty Instant Power Potion.*
4. *Ventilate and oxygenate your joints with five easy exercises and be rewarded with more youthful mobility.*
5. *Garlic is a dynamic inner cleansing food.*
6. *Dolores LaF. ended agonizing joint-muscle stiffness with the help of super-cleansing garlic.*
7. *Herbs and liniments help rub away hurtful bruises and sprains.*
8. *The R.I.C.E. remedy is beneficial for inner cleansing and pain relief.*
9. *Steam wastes out of your joints with a comfortable 30-minute warm water tub immersion.*
10. *Feed nutrients to your joints and muscles for more lasting youthful flexibility.*

Chapter 11

CLEANSE YOUR VITAL ORGANS FOR TOTAL REVITALIZATION

Wash away wastes and debris from your vital organs and experience a youthful revitalization from head to toe. With clean organs, you are able to see and hear better, enjoy a more youthful metabolism, and sing the joys of everyday living. When these organs are washed free of accumulated wastes, they function at maximum efficiency, rewarding you with strong reflexes and the look and feel of overall youth. An added bonus of cleansed organs is the freedom from discomfort, aches, disorders, and toxic-caused ailments.

DETOXIFYING YOUR EYES

In poor vision, there is nearly always some stagnation. This congestion may be due to injury to blood vessels; a too-viscid bloodstream content caused by improper nutrition and too many toxic wastes; or an improper, sluggish circulation.

Any method that improves circulation in, around, and next to the eye, can clear away congestion and improve vision or eye functions and feeling. Detoxify your eyes and you will help improve vision.

How to "Pump" Toxic Wastes Out of Your Eyes

Congestion may be relieved by a process that creates expansion and contraction of tissues within normal limits: this has a "pumping" action that improves circulation and washes out congestion. Physics teaches us that expansion is caused by heat and contraction by cold, with a few exceptions in a narrow temperature area. (Water is one of these exceptions.) You can apply this principle to your eyes, namely an application of comfortable heat and then comfortable cold to your sight organs.

You may use eye cups or clean cloths wrung out of comfortably hot water and comfortably cold water. Soak one cloth in the hot water (the heat should not cause discomfort!) and apply over the bridge of your nose, covering both closed eyes. Let this remain for five minutes. Remove. Next, take a clean cloth that has been soaked in cold water and apply over the same area for another five minutes. It is best to use two towels, one for each basin of water of differing temperatures. Continue for up to 30 minutes daily. You will help "pump" out accumulated toxic wastes that are hurtful to your sight. Your vision will be all the better with this simple remedy.

Blink Away Toxins

Blinking is instinctive, but you may not be doing it often enough to cleanse your eyes. Plan to blink frequently. It is a motion that equalizes heat energy in that area, establishing a balance between heat and coolness. Blinking washes out pollution; it is also a form of mental and eye relaxation, important to sight health. Blinking is a way of washing your eyes and keeping them clean.

Water Cleaning of Your Eyes

With the use of an eye cup (available at most health supply outlets and pharmacies), you can wash out toxins from your eyes. A few minutes of applying a water-filled eye cup (tepid or cool water) to each eye helps wash away powdery toxins from your lids and eyelashes; you will also wash off your cornea, refresh your eyes, and help improve your sight.

LESS SUGAR + LESS STRAIN = STRONGER EYESIGHT

Improve your eyesight by cutting down on sugar (source of wastes) and easing strain. Sugar and refined carbohydrates drain your body's store of chromium (a trace element needed for healthy sight). Sugar also forces your body to use its supplies of B-complex vitamins needed to regulate fluid pressure in the eyes. Refined carbohydrates deposit toxic debris in your circulatory system and block transfer of valuable sight-saving nutrients including chromium.

Eyestrain Weakens Sight

Repeated, unrelieved eyestrain from prolonged close-up visual work increases eye fluid pressure which could cause nearsightedness. If close-up work is done repeatedly, fluid pressure backs up and visual weakness is felt. *Remedy:* Every 20 minutes, change the focus of your eye and look into the distance. This back-and-forth shift helps "wash" out the blocked toxic wastes.

Toxins: Cause of Nearsightedness

An overloading of toxic wastes contributes to nearsightedness, also known as myopia. The toxemia overload changes the outward or convex curvature of the eye lens. *Explanation:* Normal eye muscles change the lens curvature constantly as you focus on objects at different distances. To focus on a nearby object, eye muscles elongate the eyeball to increase this curvature to enable light from nearby objects to focus on the retina. *Problem:* Waste accumulation leads to increased convexity which builds up more fluid pressure in the eye. *Washing Plan:* Eliminate waste-causing sugar and you limit fluid-pressure and induce an eye-washing reaction. You will then ease visual and muscular strain. You will have a chance for controlling and, hopefully, correcting nearsightedness. In brief, eliminate sugar and you "wash" your eyes.

FEED YOURSELF HEALTHIER EYESIGHT

Richard S. Kavner, O.D., who practices optometry in New York City and is former chairman of the Department of Vision Therapy at the State University of New York, urges improved nutrition for healthier vision. "Our eyes, like any other part of our body, are affected by the environment, in this case, food. And in the same way that light and pattern are nutrients for sight, vitamins and minerals are nutrients for our bodies, eyes included."

Dr. Kavner emphasizes, "The eyes are sensitive to even slight deficiencies. Depending upon the situation and the stress involved, the amount of vitamins used up by the eyes can vary widely from day to day." He offers this nutritional plan to feed yourself healthier eyesight:

1. *Vitamin A.* This substance protects against night blindness and is needed to meet the challenges of pollution, watching a lot of TV, exposure to sun glare, driving at night, and chronic eye fatigue. *Beta-carotene* is especially important; it is found in carrots, often as a yellow substance. It is transformed into vitamin A by your body, to nourish your eyes. Good sources include carrots, beet greens, parsley, watercress, broccoli, the outer leaves of lettuce, apricots, sweet potatoes, turnips, tomatoes.

2. *Vitamin B. Complex.* Important are vitamin B_1 (thiamine), B_2 (riboflavin), and B_5 (pantothenic acid). Dr. Kavner suggests getting a balance of all the B-complex vitamins and avoiding deficiencies of B_{12}, needed for red blood cell development and the nervous system. "The

B-complex vitamins are water-soluble, making them readily absorbed in the body and just as readily washed out so a new supply should be coming in daily." This family of vitamins is found in whole grains, nuts, seeds, leafy green vegetables, brewer's yeast (can be mixed into milk or fruit juices), wheat germ, and liver and eggs (but high in fat and cholesterol).

3. *Vitamin C.* Dr. Kavner says it helps keep capillaries, the tiniest blood vessels, functioning healthfully. This vitamin nourishes the lens of the eyes. "Glaucoma and cataracts are accompanied by low levels of vitamin C in the lens." In some reports, in a person weighing 150 pounds, receiving 3500 milligrams daily helps drop the intraocular pressure that causes glaucoma. "The dosage should be spaced throughout the day to protect against stomach upset." Vitamin C is found in citrus fruits such as oranges, grapefruits, lemons, and limes; in tomatoes, melons, and most vegetables (cooking lowers potency).

4. *Vitamin D.* Helps minimize myopia (nearsightedness) and protect against further deterioration. Vitamin D (with calcium) cleanses the eyes to prevent arteriosclerosis, a clogging of the arteries that interferes with blood circulation. "In the case of myopia, the vitamin D plus mineral combination appears to change the fibrous tunic surrounding the eyeball by dehydrating (cleansing) it. If this shell is water-logged, it seems to be susceptible to the pressure within and stretches into the elongated shape of a nearsighted eye. By dehydrating (cleansing) this tunic, the eyeball actually shrinks back to its more normal shape, thereby reducing the myopia. Vitamin D is available from sunshine (only 20 minutes daily) or through fortified milk, fish, egg yolk, butter, cod liver oil. (Be alert to high fat-cholesterol content of some animal foods.) Calcium is found in dairy products (low-fat or non-fat, please), green leafy vegetables, and molasses.

5. *Vitamin E.* It increases the ability of the veins and arteries to carry oxygen and cleanse pathways to the sight organs. Dr. Kavner adds, "Vitamin E appears to be extremely helpful in arresting—or even reversing—the degenerative changes in the eyes which come with old age. It has a salubrious effect on connective tissue, or collagen. When the collagen fibers of the eyes lose their elasticity, they cannot give the support needed to keep the eye from assuming an abnormal shape if other factors—such as too much near-print work—are putting stress on the eye." Dr. Kavner suggests taking vitamin E. Vitamin E is found in wheat germ, vegetable oils, whole grain cereals and breads, and leafy green vegetables.

"Remember that all vitamins and minerals work synergistically, with calcium helping D and E giving C a hand, and so on. What matters is feeling good and seeing clearly."[20]

CASE HISTORY—**Reverses Deteriorating Eyesight in Eleven Days on Easy Program**

As a machinist, Oscar T. felt his job was being jeopardized by worsening eyesight. He had to squint even at close range. His eyeglasses were exchanged for stronger and stronger lenses, even as his sight grew weaker and weaker. At times, he required help from a co-worker, who complained he "wasn't Oscar's seeing eye dog!" This cutting remark brought Oscar T. to his optometrist for help. Tests were made. Clogged waste was identified as a major problem. Also, his bloodstream showed an excessive sugar overload, together with refuse from refined starches. A mineral deficiency was also detected. Oscar T. was put on a program that eliminated refined carbohydrates, especially sugar. He boosted his intake of calcium and chromium (from supplements) and ate more raw food to clean away toxic accumulations. Almost at once, his vision became sharper. Within one week, Oscar T. could decipher tool markings without his very strong glasses. By the eleventh day, he could see rather well with milder glasses. He could read road signs and see films without eyeglasses. The simple nutritional program outlined by his optometrist had relieved his toxic-burdened eyes within a short space of time. He could then boast his restored vision was stronger than that of a guide dog!

HOW VITAMIN C + BIOFLAVONOIDS WASH AWAY CATARACT DEBRIS

Vitamin C and bioflavonoids exert a powerful cleansing process that helps wash away the grainy substances involved in the formation of cataracts. In this condition, waste accumulation increases opacity and the threat of vision loss; it is similar to a window getting frosted by cold until only the strongest light can be seen through it. To protect against this thief of sight, these two vitamins act as inner cleansers.

Vitamin C Is Protective Cleanser

This vitamin washes away debris in the lens of the eye and in the fluid directly in front of it (between lens and cornea). Vitamin C concentrated in the aqueous humor (fluid) functions as a cleanser to guard against toxic buildup involved in cataract formation.

Bioflavonoids Block Waste Corrosion

A group of nutrients that complement the cleansing action of vitamin C are the bioflavonoids. They block the accumulation of the corrosive substance, *aldose reductase*. This waste irritates components of your eyes, threatening corrosion that could predispose you to cataracts. Bioflavonoids dilute harmful wastes of *aldose reductase*, and wash it out of your aqueous humor.

Everyday Sources of Vitamin C, Bioflavonoids

These essential nutrients are found in citrus fruits (oranges, grapefruits, tangerines, lemons, limes), papaya, strawberries, cantaloupe, tomato, broccoli, green peppers, and raw leafy greens. *Important:* Vitamin C is water-soluble and perishable in air, light, and oxygen and is not stored in your body. Take in an ample supply of these foods and their juices daily. Bioflavonoids are found in highly concentrated form in the stringy portions near the rinds of citrus fruits. Plan to eat (yes, eat!) these strings when you eat the fruits. You will be giving your metabolism the needed bioflavonoids that wash away debris from your aqueous humor, thus safeguarding your vision. Supplements are available at health stores, too.

CASE HISTORY—Sight-Saving Tonic Washes Away Cataracts

Schoolteacher Minna S. was troubled with dimming vision. Blackboard writings became blurred. Identifying pupils was confusing. Fearing cataracts, she was examined by a sight specialist who said tests showed a deposit of wastes in her aqueous humor. These wastes were clouding her vision and threatening to erode segments of her eyes. He suggested a "Sight-Saving Tonic" that would introduce super-cleansing vitamin C and bioflavonoids into her system. These cleansers would wash away debris and give her sparkling clean eye fluid. They would also help eliminate *aldose reductase,* the corrosive waste involved in cataracts. Minna S. tried the tonic. Within four days, she could see better. The writing on the blackboard was sharp. She knew each pupil at a glance. At the end of six days, she had excellent vision. Gone was the threat of cataracts—they were "washed away."

How to Prepare "Sight-Saving Tonic"

Use a variety of citrus fruits, especially oranges and grapefruits, but also tangerines. Remove the peels but retain the white, string-like membrane. Add this to the fruits in a blender or electric extractor. You have a tonic that is a powerhouse of vitamin C and valuable bioflavonoids. Drink three glasses of this "Sight-Saving Tonic" daily.

Washes Debris, Boosts Sight Strength

Within moments after quaffing the tonic, the rich concentration of vitamin C along with the bioflavonoids unite to promote a super-washing of debris in your eyes. They further nourish the cells and tissues of your eyes, improving vision. They cleanse your aqueous humor so it sparkles with clean health. You see with fresh clarity, too. It is a tasty, refreshing, and sight-strengthening tonic that works swiftly.

DETOXIFYING YOUR EARS

Hearing loss is gradual. Wastes accumulate within your auditory segments, clinging together and slowly choking off the transfer of sounds. Toxemia could lead to impaired hearing. To protect against this toxic waste buildup, take advantage of effective ear-washing programs. To begin, it is helpful to know the basics about your hearing apparatus.

How Do You Hear?

Your ear is made of three main parts:

1. *Visible Outer Ear.* The outer ear is a trumpet-shaped organ with a funnel or duct that reaches to your eardrum. This is a thin, tautly stretched membrane which vibrates when struck by sound waves.
2. *Middle Ear.* On the opposite side of the eardrum is your middle ear, which contains three small bones shaped like a hammer, anvil, and stirrup. When sound waves make the ear drum vibrate, this sound is transported along the three small bones and then into the fluid of your inner ear.
3. *Inner Ear.* In the cochlea, the hearing organ of the inner ear, there are tiny, electrically charged hairs that bend and flex in response to sound. They carry an electric-like current through the nerve of hearing to the brain. Your inner ear also contains a fluid that bathes these hairs and keeps them clean and alert. These microscopic hairs move back and forth, conducting sound waves to the hearing nerve, which then transmits it electrically to your brain.

Clean Membrane—Sharper Hearing

When your inner ear is kept clear of debris, it receives more vibrations through the eardrum. You should then be able to hear sound frequencies of about 25,000 cycles per second. You will hear with youthful acuity. *Problem:* When debris covers your membrane, when wastes clog up your inner ear fluids and become waste puddles, you begin to suffer hearing loss. Deafness might be said to begin, in part, by a viscid condition of the blood, lymph, and interstitial spaces (between cells and tissues) because of accumulation of toxins. There is congestion of small capillaries; the mucous lining of the body is suffused. Viscid wastes are "dumped" or even "stored" in parts of your ear. This is especially dangerous in your eustachian tube (the tube that connects the middle ear to the pharynx; it allows pressure on the inner side of the eardrum to remain equal to the external pressure). The eustachian tube becomes clogged with adhesions or toxic wastes. This sticky congestion spreads through the tube into the vestibule of the ear and hearing problems strike.

To correct this hearing threat, cleanse the debris clogging up your ear membrane and fluids.

HOW TO CLEANSE AND ENERGIZE YOUR EARS FOR SUPER-HEARING

If you eat excessive amounts of refined carbohydrates (sugars and starches) you cause a speedy jump in your blood sugar. Moments later, the blood sugar plunges. This causes an up-and-down insulin "yank." It has its repercussions on your hearing.

Problem

Your inner ear has one of the highest needs for energy, as compared to other organs. An up-and-down blood sugar yank pours excessive wastes or "fallout" from refined foods onto your membranes and fluids. This shift constricts the highly sensitive vascular network in your ears. They become "energy-starved." Oxygen is choked off. Nutrients cannot reach your ears. Circulation is blocked. Wastes build up. Your hearing starts to deteriorate. *Speedy Solution:* Eliminate refined, processed, and chemically treated foods. Avoid refined carbohydrate foods. Switch to fresh fruits, vegetables, legumes, and whole grains. Lean meat products may be eaten in moderation.

Inner Cleansing Benefits: These foods are prime sources of vitamin A, needed to nourish and cleanse the sensory receptor cells of the inner ears. They supply B-complex vitamins to balance blood sugar metabolism; they also cleanse the nerves of your hearing components. Vitamin C scrubs away wastes, cleans the membrane, washes debris from the fluids in your inner ears, and then scrubs clean the microscopic hairs.

Within moments, hearing becomes improved. You enjoy better sound transmission. You no longer miss words, or have to cup your ear to listen to normal conversational levels or keep asking, "What did you say?" Cleanse your hearing from *within* on this detoxification program and you speedily energize your ears for super-hearing from *without*.

THE LOW-FAT WAY TO IMPROVED HEARING

Reduce intake of hard animal fats. They glue together red blood cells, choking off the flow of oxygen to your inner ears. Elevated blood levels of fat attract wastes that erect blockages to interfere with hearing. You need to make an important nutritional change.

More Vegetable Fats for Better Hearing

Make a switch. Use free flowing oils and unhydrogenated fats (those that are liquid at room temperature). Limit or eliminate hard animal fats. Of course, use oils in moderation. Don't go overboard since they, too, are fats, albeit safer than the hard fats. A few tablespoons a day is your limit as replacement for hard fat. You'll help clean your cells and wash out toxic blockages that threaten your hearing.

CASE HISTORY—From "Nearly Deaf" to "Total Hearing" in Sixteen Days

As a sales manager, Benedict U. had to be a good listener as much as a good talker. When he began to "miss" words or, worse, "misunderstand" what customers and supervisors said, he became worried. Gradually, his hearing diminished until he feared something worse than job loss: isolation from the world! He was examined by an audiologist (hearing specialist) who diagnosed an overlayer of waste material clogging his hearing apparatus. Too many hard fats had glued together his red blood cells. Too many refined foods played havoc with his blood sugar, and his hearing was "choked" off. Benedict U. was put on a program of natural, low-fat foods. His detoxified hearing components made sound transmission as clear as the proverbial bell.

DETOXIFYING YOUR KIDNEYS

Your kidneys are your body's filter plant, through which over 150 quarts of fluid pass daily. They are situated at the back of your abdomen, below the diaphragm, one on each side of the spine. These two large organs filter your bloodstream and remove impurities.

Each kidney consists of a million tiny filters that remove wastes from your blood, dilute them in water, and then excrete them via urine. Blood enters one end of each tiny kidney tube and is propelled through the other (smaller) end. This should be an effective filtering process, but if toxic wastes accumulate, the blood becomes clogged. The risk of uremic poisoning looms.

Simple Water Drinking Washes Away Kidney Debris

Accumulated debris may cling together to form kidney stones. These are crystallized bits of wastes that back up in the kidneys. Most kidney stones consist of urates, phosphates, oxalates, and other wastes that cling to your vital organs. You want to break down and wash away these toxins. Simple water drinking is an amazing remedy.

Washes, Cleanses, Detoxifies

The water you drink becomes part of your bloodstream; it works to wash away wastes, cleanse your kidneys, detoxify your kidney tubes. Water dilutes the small, irritating, burr-like clumps that hook together and threaten to form into kidney stones. *Remedy:* Daily quaffing of fresh water regulates your temperature, lubricates your joints and muscles, improves digestion, and facilitates the washing out of wastes from your kidneys and entire body, too. It is the refreshing, rejuvenating remedy for healthy organs.

CASE HISTORY—Drinks Away Kidney Wastes in Short Time

Toxic accumulation made Brenda O'R. feel sluggish. She was troubled with a sour stomach and disposition to match! Her internist said she was "dehydrated" because she did not drink enough water daily. Diagnosis: kidney wastes that clumped together and could form stones requiring surgery. Anxious to avoid the knife, she followed the internist's amazingly simple program—drink six to eight glasses of water daily. Immediately, Brenda O'R. felt a clearing up of her sluggishness. In four days, she felt more alert, more energetic. In six days, she was cheerful in body, mind, and attitude. Her internist confirmed her hopes. The wastes had been washed away. She was saved from the threat of surgery . . . thanks to drinking water!

Other Sources of Detoxifying Liquid

Fresh fruit and vegetable juices are good sources of detoxifying liquids. Also, plant foods as part of a salad also have high natural water content together with healthy nutrients. Herbal teas, salt-free soups, and salt-free seltzer all help detoxify your system with an abundant supply of liquid.

THE BERRY JUICE THAT DISSOLVES KIDNEY GRAVEL

Cranberry juice is an excellent source of vitamin C and contains a natural fruit acid that reportedly dissolves gravel in the kidneys and washes it out of your body. The acid soil of New England which nurtures and nourishes the cranberry, gives to it the same detoxifying power that boosts kidney cleansing.

Drink Cranberry Juice

Just two or three glasses of cranberry juice delivers a highly concentrated and potent acid to dissolve the gravel. If the juice is too tart, add a little apple juice and a bit of honey. *Cleansing Benefit:* The vitamin C and the cranberry acid break up oxalate clumps and speeds their removal through waste channels. It's a tasty and refreshing way to keep your kidneys clean and your body in youthful shape, too.

Keep Away From Oxalate-Containing Foods

Oxalate is a substance found in many foods. Usually, it combines with calcium in the digestive tract and is given off as calcium oxalate. But if you have a fat malabsorption disorder, the fat you eat will combine with the calcium in foods and both are excreted. But, the oxalate is left free of calcium and cannot be passed off; it is absorbed in your system. Since the oxalate cannot be broken down in your body, it goes to your kidneys for excretion into the urine. But in your kidneys, the oxalate joins with calcium to form calcium oxalate stones. This is the risk! You need to reduce or restrict oxalate-rich foods.

High Oxalate Foods

baked beans in tomato sauce	chocolate and cocoa
mustard greens	spinach
okra	black tea
beets	eggplant

Go Easy on Protein

Protein increases the acidity of urine, but it also accelerates the presence of uric acid which could lead to the formation of stones.

Vitamin B$_6$ (Pyridoxine) Has Cleansing Action

This vitamin helps control your body's production of oxalate, while prompting a waste-cleansing action. It is found in whole grain breads, cereals, bananas, nuts, potatoes; also in poultry and liver, but watch the fat-cholesterol content.

DETOXIFYING YOUR LIVER

Your liver performs many functions essential to your life and wellbeing. Located behind the lower ribs on the right side of your abdomen, it weighs about three pounds and is roughly the size of a football.

Liver Functions

Basically your liver (1) converts food into nutrients necessary for life and growth; (2) manufactures and exports important substances used by the rest of your body; (3) detoxifies and eliminates substances that would otherwise be poisonous. In essence, your liver is your body's refinery. It plays the principal role in removing from your blood both ingested and internally produced toxic substances. It also makes bile, a bitter yellow-green fluid which is essential for digestion. Bile is stored in your gallbladder, which contracts after eating and discharges bile into your intestine to help digestion.

Waste Backup Leads to Liver Distress

Waste accumulation hampers proper filtering by your liver and leads to such disorders as skin discoloration (jaundice), cirrhosis (scarring), abdominal swelling, fatigue, and nausea. These symptoms suggest inner cleansing is needed.

Guidelines for Keeping Your Liver Clean

Avoid all forms of salt, sugar, and irritating seasonings. Avoid white flour products, commercial cereals, processed or artificially preserved foods, soft drinks, alcohol, tobacco, fatty and fried foods, rancid oils.

How to Protect Your Liver From Toxic Overload

Avoid alcohol. It is a common toxin that both attacks and is metabolized by your liver. Heavy drinkers often develop hepatitis, an inflammation of the liver causing irregular bile flow. This condition may progress to cirrhosis, a fatty overgrowth of the tissues with accompanying degeneration of the cells. When your liver ceases to function so does your body! Be cautious about mixing medications; in particular, alcohol and many "over-the-counter" and prescription medicines do not mix well.

Fluid retention (edema) may be decreased by a diet restricted in salt. Toxins which accumulate in your body are the result of bacterial action on excessive protein. A decrease in dietary protein would result in less toxin formation.

Laxatives which speed up the movement of proteins through the

Digestive System

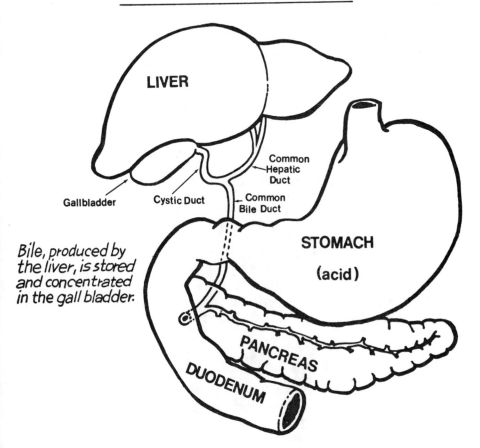

LIVER

Common Hepatic Duct

Common Bile Duct

Gallbladder

Cystic Duct

STOMACH

(acid)

Bile, produced by the liver, is stored and concentrated in the gall bladder.

PANCREAS

DUODENUM

gastrointestinal system, could be habit forming. Switch to a high-fiber, raw food program for more natural inner cleansing.

At the same time, enjoy lots of exercise, fresh air, and rest. This improves your total body health. You'll feel refreshed, cleansed, and remade all over, thanks to a detoxified liver.

HOW TO DETOXIFY YOUR GALLBLADDER

Your gallbladder is a small, pear-shaped organ that averages three to six inches in length. It is tucked under the liver and is connected to the liver and intestine by small tubes called bile ducts. Bile is the fluid essential to the digestion of fatty foods; it is produced by the liver and secreted into the gallbladder which serves as a receptacle for the concentration and storage of bile.

When food is eaten and prepared for assimilation, a tube from your gallbladder opens to let the bile pour into your intestine to metabolize the food. If your gallbladder cannot function properly, then fragments of improperly digested food cause waste accumulation.

Toxemia Wastes Form Into Gallstones

When the bile becomes too congested with sludge, the fat precipitates into crystals that form stones. These vary in size from small pebbles to stones as large as golf balls. Sometimes, these stones become stuck in the bile ducts leading from the gallbladder to the duodenum (first part of small intestine). The gallbladder and bile ducts then try to push the stones out by muscular contractions. This can cause attacks of excruciating abdominal pain. Blockage of the ducts by stones also prevents flow of bile into the intestines. Bile then backs up into the bloodstream, causing jaundice. This is one penalty of toxin overload.

Basic Inner Cleansing Plan

In any type of gallbladder disturbance, your diet should be low in fat, especially animal fat. You may not be able to tolerate spices, condiments, coffee, strong-flavored cooked vegetables, or eggs. All fried foods and pastries should be avoided. You'll help promote inner cleansing with these basic guidelines.

THE FOOD THAT WASHES AWAY GALLBLADDER WASTES

Taken from soybeans or sunflower seeds, lecithin promotes a gallbladder scrubbing action that may well wash away stone-forming toxic wastes. Lecithin is a soap-like food that can emulsify fats and dissolve water-soluble substances at the same time. Lecithin breaks down the precipitated cholesterol that is often part of the gallstones. Lecithin prompts the manufacture of *cholic acid,* a natural scrubbing substance found in bile. Lecithin urges cholic acid to attack the precipitated cholesterol crystals and break them down for elimination.

Lecithin is also a source of phospholipids which prevent cholesterol fats from clumping together. There are two major types of gallstones. *Cholesterol gallstones,* composed mainly of cholesterol, account for almost 80 percent of all cases. *Pigment gallstones,* composed mainly of calcium salts of bile pigments and other compounds, account for the remaining 20 percent. Therefore, since most have cholesterol gallstones, the use of lecithin is advantageous for inner cleansing. Lecithin breaks down the accumulations and frees the bladder from these glue-like encumbrances. Lecithin may well be the one food that washes away gallbladder toxins.

Easy Use of Lecithin

Sprinkle two or three tablespoons of granules daily (from health store) onto raw salads. They are great with your breakfast cereal, or add to soups, stews, casseroles, and baked goods. In a hurry? Add two teaspoons to a tall glass of vegetable juice. Stir vigorously (or blenderize) and enjoy!

PLAIN WATER HELPS WASH AWAY GALLBLADDER CRYSTALS

Drinking up to six glasses of plain water or other natural liquids daily will help liquefy the crystals and wash the grit right out of your eliminative channels. Throughout the day, drink this natural source of inner cleansing. Water keeps your body as clean and sparkling fresh as itself!

CASE HISTORY—Gallbladder Crystals Break Up, Wash Out of Body

Middle-aged Carole L. feared she would follow in the footsteps of her older sisters who endured much pain and underwent gallbladder removal. She felt frequent spasms, indigestion, chills, and fever. She was concerned about her sagging skin. Was she destined for surgery? She discussed it with her prevention-oriented holistic physician. He examined her carefully, then prescribed the lecithin plan and at least six glasses of water daily. Carole L. followed the program. Almost at once, the pain and discomfort ended. Her skin perked up. A future examination brought the good news that she was out of danger of stone formation. Carole L. had been able to break up (thanks to lecithin) and wash out (thanks to pure water) the accumulated toxic wastes—all in a matter of two weeks.

Keeping Your Gallbladder Free of Toxins

Follow the general inner cleansing guidelines outlined throughout this book. Avoid hard animal fats as much as possible. Boost intake of fresh fruits, vegetables, whole grains, legumes, nuts, and seeds. Drink lots of water and freshly prepared juices. Lose excess weight. Keep cholesterol under control. Gallbladder toxemia is twice as common in women as in men, so women should be more prudent in following inner cleansing and detoxification programs. *Tip:* Increase your fiber intake. Fiber not only helps prevent constipation and diverticulosis, it appears to help prevent the formation of gallstones. About 30 grams of fiber daily will give you that cleansing benefit.

You can enjoy a feeling of detoxification when you have sparkling clean organs. Free them of debris and glue-like wastes, and you will discover what a wonderful joy life can be.

─────────── *HIGHLIGHTS* ───────────

1. *Wash away wastes and improve your eyesight on a sugar-free and refined carbohydrate-free program. Nutrition is recommended by a doctor for feeding your eyes.*

2. *Oscar T. reversed his deteriorating eyesight in eleven days on a simple detoxification plan.*

3. *Vitamin C plus bioflavonoids wash away cataract-threatening debris.*

4. *Schoolteacher Minna S. used the delicious "Sight-Saving Tonic" to save her eyes from surgery.*

5. *Sharpen your hearing with an improved nutritional program. It calls for less animal fats for cleaner ears and better hearing.*

6. *Benedict U. went from "nearly deaf" to "total hearing" in two weeks on a simple detoxification plan.*

7. *Brenda O'R. was able to wash and cleanse her kidneys with water.*

8. *Cranberry juice is a tangy way to dissolve kidney gravel.*

9. *Lecithin has a scrubbing action on your bladder to cleanse it of toxic wastes.*

10. *Carole L. followed a lecithin and water detoxification plan that ended her gallbladder distress.*

Chapter 12

HOW TO CLEANSE YOUR BLOODSTREAM AND ENRICH YOUR ENTIRE BODY

The cleaner your bloodstream, the healthier your body. When you realize that every part of your body is bathed, washed, nourished, and oxygenated by your bloodstream around-the-clock, you understand the importance of having a clean "river of life." You need a rich supply of red blood cells to deposit essential nutrients on your vital organs and trillions of cells. This is your very foundation of inner rejuvenation. To free yourself from internal pollution, clean up your bloodstream.

Continuous Process Requires Rich Blood

Your circulatory system is responsible for: the uninterrupted delivery of oxygenated blood and its nutrients to your trillions of tissue cells; their exchange for waste products of metabolism; the transportation of wastes to points of elimination. Hardly any other body system has such a great responsibility as your circulatory system. Without a supply of clean, oxygenated blood, your tissues and cells would soon die. To keep them not only alive, but throbbing with youthful vitality, you need rich, clean blood.

Blood Sediment Causes Ill Health

As blood flows through your circulatory system, it picks up waste products left through oxidation and is responsible for their elimination. During this process, the waste products are passed through the microscopically thin walls of your capillaries (tiny blood vessels). It is inevitable for some sediment to remain behind. If there is a brief spell of sluggishness, more waste remains in the bloodstream instead of being discharged through your capillaries. Incomplete metabolism leaves behind fragments and bits of refuse in your bloodstream. If allowed to build up, such sediment can choke off your free-flowing blood circulation and impair your health. You need to keep your

153

blood clean with simple, effective home washing programs. Let's see how you can do this promptly.

THE EVERYDAY FOOD THAT CREATES A SPARKLING CLEAN BLOODSTREAM

Remove the most stubborn sludge deposits from your blood and be rewarded with a sparkling clean bloodstream. You can do it with an everyday food—garlic. This amazing vegetable is able to initiate the synthesis or the breakdown of waste substances that stubbornly cling to your red and white blood cells. Garlic dissolves these wastes and propels them toward your eliminative channels. It is a powerful blood cleanser.

Two Powerful Blood Cleaning Substances in Garlic

Almost instantly after you consume garlic, your digestive system metabolizes two of its most powerful cleansers, propyldisulfide and diallyldisulfide. In combination, they swirl through your circulatory system, acting like magnets in attracting wastes, uprooting sludge deposits, breaking down stubborn clumps, and swiftly washing them out of your body. This super-cleansing action occurs within minutes after you consume garlic. It is a dynamic blood washer.

One Garlic Clove a Day Keeps Your Bloodstream Clean

You may have more than this amount, of course, but the minimum is one clove per day. You may add a finely chopped garlic clove (or more) to a plate of raw vegetables. You could also have garlic juice. Use a garlic press (from health stores or housewares outlets) and squeeze drops of juice from several cloves into a glass of vegetable juice. Stir vigorously and drink before your main meal. You could also add a few chopped garlic cloves to a stew, soup, casserole, or any baked dish. Daily intake of garlic will be introducing a powerful "dirt magnet" into your bloodstream that gathers up sludge and then whirls it out of your body. A cleaner bloodstream is your reward.

CASE HISTORY—Corrects Cold Hands, Feet, Constant Chills in Two Days

Marcia J.H. would wear sweaters and gloves in the warmest weather. As a computer programmer, she complained of cold working conditions even when the heat was turned on at top levels. Marcia J.H. shivered even if she sat in the warm sun. A company registered nurse took some tests and said

Marcia J.H. had "unclean blood," which sounded as unpleasant as it felt! The nurse suggested she consume at least three garlic cloves daily with her regular meals to detoxify her sludge-filled blood. Toxic waste blockages choked her bloodstream and it could not provide warming oxygenated nourishment to her cells and organs. This was the root cause of her constant "ice cold" feeling even in warm weather.

Marcia J.H. followed the program. Immediately, she experienced a throbbing vitality. In two days, she was so warm, she glowed with a radiant complexion and discarded her sweater and gloves. She even complained that the department in which she worked was too warm. Garlic had warmed her body by cleansing her bloodstream in only two days.

IRON—THE MINERAL THAT REJUVENATES YOUR BLOOD

Wake up your tired blood with iron! It energizes your body by cleansing your bloodstream and performing lifegiving functions such as:

- Transferring oxygen and carbon dioxide to and from body tissues.
- Assisting in the synthesis of heme iron in immature and sludge-burdened red blood cells. Heme iron combines with protein to form hemoglobin, the red pigment in blood that carries oxygen.
- Transforming beta-carotene into vitamin A for inner cleansing.
- Helping form purines as part of nucleic acids.
- Removing fats from your bloodstream.
- Assisting in the synthesis of collagen, the protein that binds cells together.
- Helping produce antibodies that fight off infectious invaders and clean your cells.
- Helping produce enzymes that are involved in releasing energy from your cells.

Hemoglobin, Sludge, Anemia, Fatigue

Hemoglobin, the component in red blood cells that provides them with their rich red color, brings energy-giving oxygen to every body cell. But when excessive sludge and toxemia push hemoglobin levels below normal, your cells become choked with wastes. They are deprived of oxygen. Result: energy-zapping anemia—and fatigue!

Toxemia to Blame For Tired Blood

Your body's capacity to carry cleansing oxygen plummets because of low levels of iron and other nutrients. Toxemia increases. You have "tired blood" when you have these symptoms: excessive fatigue, palpitations, shortness of breath, marked pallor of skin and nail beds, "pins and needles" or numbness in your extremities. Headaches and gastrointestinal problems are additional reactions to toxic wastes in your bloodstream. If neglected, you have unexplained and persistent fatigue, unusual irritability, reduced work performance, poor concentration, and unusual sensitivity to cold.

Women Need More Iron On a Daily Basis

"The active woman requires more of certain dietary components than their sedentary neighbors," says Joan Ullyot, M.D., sports medicine specialist of San Francisco, California. "Extra iron is a must! This is especially important in active women because of the high oxygen demand. Iron carries and binds oxygen in blood and muscles. One food supplement I recommend for all women who are still menstruating is iron. The American diet does not contain enough iron to replace what is lost. Even if you eat oodles of liver, spinach, and egg yolks, all iron-rich foods, you'll barely manage to keep up. And there may be added iron loss in active women through perspiration."

Dr. Ullyot emphasizes, "Iron deficiency is extremely noticeable in active women because of high oxygen demands of physical exertion. If you have an unexplained slump in your performance, it may be due to a sudden iron deficiency."

How Much Daily Iron?

Dr. Ullyot answers, "I strongly advise supplementing your diet with at least a 'multi-vitamin with iron' compound. These usually contain 18 to 30 milligrams of iron. The average replacement requirement per day to make up for menstrual loss is two milligrams. This represents the normal 10 percent absorption of 20 milligrams in the diet."[21]

Iron in Your Food

Iron is available in two forms: (1) heme iron, found only in foods of animal origin; (2) nonheme iron, found in both animal and vegetable sources. While liver and red meats are potent iron sources, they are also high in saturated fat, cholesterol, and calories. *Suggestion:* Strike a balance! Eat meat on occasion, then fill out your iron needs with iron-rich plant foods. See the following chart.

SOURCES OF IRON

Food	Amount	Iron (mg)
*Cereals, cold, ready-to-eat	1 cup	18.0
Oatmeal, hot, 100% iron-fortified	⅓ cup	18.0
Liver, beef, braised	⅓ cup	18.0
Prune juice	8 oz.	10.4
Apricots, dried	1 cup	7.2
Molasses, blackstrap	2 tbsp.	6.4
Beef, lean cuts	3 oz.	2.5
Lima beans, dry, cooked	1 cup	6.0
Beans, red kidney and white, cooked	1 cup	4.6
Lentils, cooked	1 cup	4.2
Tofu	1 cup	4.2
Peas, fresh or frozen, cooked	1 cup	3.0
Wheat germ	2 tbsp.	2.8
Turkey, roasted, white meat, skinless	7 oz.	2.8

*Iron content of cereals varies by brand and flavor. Read package label.

Plan a Variety of Iron Foods

While your body best absorbs iron from animal products, try vegetable sources: beans, dark leafy greens, peas—great detoxification foods. You may want to mix in a bit of fish or poultry at the same meal, but this is optional.

If You Use a Supplement

Read the label to see you are not getting excessive amounts of iron. Keep within the U.S. Recommended Daily Allowance of 18 milligrams for women 15 to 50 years of age; 10 milligrams for women over 50. For some, ferrous fumarate may be less irritable to the digestive tract and more easily absorbed.

HOW TO PUMP IRON INTO YOUR BLOODSTREAM

To invigorate iron absorption, try these low-fat, low-calorie tips for boosting assimilation:

Have Lots of Vitamin C

It increases absorption of nonheme iron. At the same meal, include iron-rich foods together with vitamin C foods such as citrus fruit or juice, strawberries, tomatoes, melons, potatoes, cabbage, cantaloupe, and dark-green vegetables.

Use Cast-Iron Pots, Pans, Skillets and Utensils

When acidic foods (tomato sauce, for example) are cooked in these iron pans, some of the iron enters the food, boosting its iron content. Plan to use an acidic food when cooking an iron-containing food in a cast-iron pot or pan.

Avoid Coffee and Tea

Caffeine and other substances in these beverages greatly decrease iron absorption. Switch to herbal teas or fruit or vegetable juices (for vitamin C, too).

Preserve Nutrients In Foods

Use the least amount of heat and water and minimum cooking time. *Tip:* Maintain nutrient power if you steam vegetables rather than boil them. Tastier, too.

Eating High-Fiber Foods?

Be sure you have an abundant amount of iron. Bran and other substances in fiber interfere with iron absorption.

All-Natural Iron Cocktail

Combine 1 tablespoon of blackstrap molasses with 8 ounces of orange juice. Stir vigorously or blenderize for two minutes. Enjoy! (A powerhouse with both iron and vitamin C working in combination to nourish your red cells and give them super-scrubbing power.)

HOW TO WASH AND "IRON" YOUR BLOOD CELLS FOR SUPER HEALTH

Put more life into your body with washed and "ironed" blood cells. This does not refer to any laundering iron, but rather to a "cell washing" first and a "cell nourishing" second with the use *of iron,* the amazing nutrient. It has the power to invigorate your blood cells, to give you the look and feel of super health. You can "wash out" and "iron-nourish" your blood cells in a simple two-part program. Here's how.

First: Cell-Washing

Uproot the accumulated blood sediment and prepare it for elimination by opening your skin pores to steam out these toxic wastes. You do this in a simple and refreshing *contrast bath*. It takes 20 minutes and gives you a feeling of youthfulness by cleaning your bloodstream. Follow these easy steps.

1. Fill your bathtub with water warm enough to create clouds of steam. It should be comfortable but not burning, of course.

2. Immerse yourself. Luxuriate in the steaming warmth for 15 minutes. You should perspire. You can see the uprooted sediment being washed out of your blood and body cells.

3. Let the water run out of the tub. Stand up. (Careful! Hold on to a bar to avoid skidding.) Turn on a needle-spray cool shower. It should give you a pleasant (not hurtful) sting. This washes away the steamed-out sediment. The cool water closes your pores, protecting you against incoming pollutants. Less than three minutes of this contrasting shower is all you need.

5. Step on a non-skid bath mat. Dry yourself with a rough towel. You have steamed out impurities and will experience the reward of an invigorated bloodstream.

Second: Cell-Ironing

The second step of this two-part "wash and iron" blood cell program calls for nutrition. You need to feed the breath of life to your cells by giving them *iron*. This nutrient helps produce *hemoglobin,* the red coloring matter of your cells. Iron further increases and invigorates the manufacture of your white blood cells. Called *leukocytes,* they are somewhat larger than the red cells. They have the lifesaving power of destroying toxic invaders. But these white blood cells are not permanent. They wear out, break down, disintegrate. If not replaced, they could become deficient, which means the sediment and wastes will accumulate. If improperly cleansed, these wastes stick together. They form blockages which interfere with free-flowing blood circulation. To boost the restoration and vigor of leukocytes that cleanse toxic wastes, feed them iron with this "cell-ironing" (iron-feeding) program:

1. Boost intake of these high iron-rich foods: fish, whole grain cereals and breads, dark leafy green vegetables, sun-dried fruits such as apricots, raisins, prunes, dates.

2. Combine iron foods together with a vitamin C food. The iron is best absorbed when energized with the backup of vitamin C *at the same time*. This iron-feeding plan will give an exhilarating rejuvenation to your white cells. Within moments, these foods scour your bloodstream, cleanse away debris, and make you feel warm and alive all over. This combination works almost immediately. Tasty, too.

3. Take one to two tablespoons of blackstrap molasses with any favorite fruit juice daily. This gives you a high concentration of iron *together* with vitamin C—A dynamic energizer to your blood-cleansing white cells.

4. Daily, take the following "C + Iron Tonic" to immediately regenerate your trillions of waste-washing white blood cells.

C + Iron Tonic

In a glass of fresh citrus juice, add one tablespoon of blackstrap molasses, several teaspoons of sun-dried fruits. Blenderize for 60 seconds. Drink this "C + Iron Tonic" daily before your main meal. It is a powerhouse of cell rejuvenation and blood cleansing.

CASE HISTORY—**Restored to Life With C + Iron Tonic**

Jennifer W.M. was troubled with shortness of breath. Her hands trembled. Her eyes looked dull. She had that aged, wizened appearance that made her look much older than 45. Family and friends worried she was aging rapidly. Jennifer W.M. was advised to boost intake of iron foods and supplements. She did, but the benefits were still negligible. Something was wrong. Her hematologist (blood specialist) diagnosed her condition as a scarcity of blood-washing white cells. The iron in the foods she was eating was not being fully absorbed because it lacked enough vitamin C at the same time. He told her to take the "C + Iron Tonic" daily. This *combination* would revitalize her metabolism. The iron would be absorbed fully to energize her white cells to scour and cleanse her bloodstream. Within three days, Jennifer W.M. revived. She breathed easily. Her hands were steady (warm, too), and her eyes sparkled. She walked and acted with the vitality of a young woman. She felt she had been "restored to life" with the help of this cell-scrubbing C + Iron Tonic.

BALLOON BREATHING BUILDS STRONGER BLOOD CELLS

What You Need

You'll need a simple balloon. Get the very thick kind that calls for much strenuous blowing.

How to Do It

Breathe in through your nose. Fill your lungs. Blow air into the balloon until it is filled. Relax and let the air out of the balloon, then repeat. Plan to balloon breathe a full ten minutes daily. Gradually, increase to fifteen minutes.

Cellular Cleansing Benefits

The deep inhalation floods your 750 million air sacs with oxygen. The oxygen travels through the cells to get into your bloodstream. Your red and white blood cells now absorb the oxygen and use it for self-regeneration. The oxygenated blood cells work swiftly (the air revived and energized them) to cleanse away stagnant clumps blocking your bloodstream. Within moments, the blood washing process detoxifies your system, thanks to the "fun" way of oxygenating your circulatory system.

CASE HISTORY—Inhalation Programs Create New Will to Live

Walking with a stooped posture, bleary-eyed, Will D.E. was aging at an alarming rate. A consulting engineer, he found it difficult to concentrate on blueprints. He became confused with the simplest of mechanical terms. His professional status was jeopardized by his declining health. He felt so drained, at times he said he had no desire to continue on. It was as if he had lost the will to live.

A physiotherapist suggested he revive his bloodstream with a simple inhalation program. It would bring welcome nourishing oxygen to his air-starved blood cells. Within moments, the alerted cells would perform the needed debris-sweeping and waste-washing functions. Desperate, Will D.E. followed the inhalation program. He did the deep breathing and the balloon routine. Almost at once, he felt himself revive. His posture improved, his face perked up, he looked younger. In three days on this cellular oxygenation program, he bounced back with renewed vigor. His cleansed bloodstream made him sparkle with the joy of life. All this through easy (and free) inhalation! Now he had a new will to live!

Healthy red blood cells contain sufficient hemoglobin which gives blood its color and carries detoxifying oxygen through the body. You may not see your bloodstream, but you can feel the rewards of having it washed when you experience that "great to be alive" feeling that comes with this cleansing. With the help of nutrition, water, and inhalation, you can revitalize your bloodstream and entire body.

────────────────── *HIGHLIGHTS* ──────────────────

1. *Garlic is a concentrated source of two blood cleansers that make it a powerful detoxifying food.*

2. *Marcia J.H. corrected body chills by cleaning her blood with garlic.*

3. *Wash and "iron" your bloodstream with the simple, two-part program, in the privacy of your home—in less than 30 minutes.*

4. *Check the list of iron foods and learn how to get the most power out of this mineral.*

5. *For top-notch washing, combine vitamin C plus iron in the life restoring "C + Iron Tonic." It made Jennifer W.M. become alive again.*

6. *Oxygenate your tired blood cells and improve their cleansing power in minutes. Try the fun-filled balloon breathing program, too. This inhalation program gave Will D.E. a new "will to live."*

Chapter 13

CLEANSE YOUR ARTERIES AND ENJOY A "SECOND YOUTH"

Clean debris from your arteries and immediately experience the joy of "second youth" from head to toe. Your arteries are elastic tubes. Their task is to carry oxygen-reinforced fresh blood from your heart to all parts of your body. To carry out this rejuvenating-nourishing inner cleansing, they must be kept as free of sediment as possible. Only then will they maintain this vital total body nourishment for the look and feel of youthful health. A problem occurs when errors in daily living deposit wastes in your body's "pipelines," posing a risk to your youthful health.

WASTE OVERLOAD = CLOGGED ARTERIES

Wastes from incompletely metabolized byproducts of undesirable foods accumulate on the insides of artery walls. These wastes sneakily form into fatty deposits. Such sludge gradually becomes thicker and thicker. More deposits are attracted. As the waste overload continues, the inside walls of your arteries become so clogged, the blood cannot move along at a normal rate. The space inside the arteries grows smaller. More pressure is exerted on the blood. This waste overload poses a serious health threat.

Danger Symptoms

Clogged arteries with choking fatty deposits cause symptoms such as cramps or tingling, sharp aches or pains when you move arms or legs. Emotional disorders such as memory lapses and fuzzy thinking are blamed on wastes that have accumulated on arteries leading to your brain. Your vital organs (heart, kidneys, liver) react when wastes gather on arteries leading to these areas. When these organs are denied adequate blood-bearing nourishment because of waste-choked arteries, they become ill. So does the rest of you.

Prolonged Sediment Buildup Threatens Life

As more and more sediment collects on the walls of your arteries, the risk of the sediment expanding into your bloodstream and forming a life-threatening blockage increases. These wastes may break off in chunks and float around in your blood. If the wastes float toward a smaller blood vessel, they become lodged between the walls. This can lead to a serious stroke that may be crippling or fatal! Be alert—prolonged sediment accumulation on and within your arteries presents a dangerous threat to your life.

ARTERIOSCLEROSIS—EXCESS SLUDGE BUILDUP

In this condition, there is a slow pileup of wastes. The arteries become narrow and hard. They lose their flexibility. There is a buildup of plaques in the arterial walls, which may cause an occlusion (literally, a cutting off) of blood flow. This is the forerunner of a crippling form of coronary artery disease.

Neglect Worsens Problem

A typical plaque may break apart. It then spews out dead wastes and sludge into the artery. This upsets the blood flow, forcing platelets to accumulate at the site of the breakage. These stick to each other and to the wall to fill the channel. Parts of half-formed thrombi (waste accumulations) may break loose from the wall and lodge in a plaque-narrowed part of the artery.

The arterial wall, weakened by formation of dense plaques, may bulge and bleed (an aneurysm, or a ballooning-out at the wall of a blood vessel) or burst completely. Spasms, a temporary closing of the blood vessels, become a new threat. Your life is at serious risk as the waste sludge accumulates until it chokes off your blood circulation. Without delay, you need to have clean arteries—they are the very lifeline of youthful health.

CAN FOOD MAKE YOU FEEL YOUNG FOREVER?

Certain everyday foods have the power to clean your arteries and help you feel young forever. This is the discovery made by Julian Whitaker, M.D., director of the California (San Clemente) Health Treatment Center. He finds that a high-carbohydrate, low-fat food program promotes cleansing to heal many "incurable" ailments to give you many years of feeling young and active.

Basic Program

"My patients are put on a supervised program in which complex carbohydrates make up 80 percent of their calorie intake. The balance is made up of low-fat, low-cholesterol, and low-protein foods." *Note:* Complex carbohydrates are abundant in whole grain breads and cereals, corn, potatoes, and especially fresh fruits and vegetables and legumes.

Improves Heart Health

Dr. Whitaker labels fat as a villain in heart health and blames it for waste overload. "When large amounts of fat are eaten, the red blood cells stick together and stack up. This sludge is called *rouleaux formation* which limits the flow of blood cells through the capillaries. It creates 'sludging' with a 30 percent reduction of oxygen supply to the heart." The doctor prescribes a low-fat program as a means of boosting better oxygen supply to nourish the heart. This promotes a "forever young" feeling of overall health.

Arteriosclerosis and Cholesterol

"Clogged arteries may eventually be reversed by reducing fat intake in your diet. Cholesterol levels can be brought down 30 to 40 percent so your risk of heart disease may be reduced and eliminated." *Simple Plan:* Dr. Whitaker accomplishes arterial cleansing by putting his patients on a higher whole grain and natural carbohydrate food program—but with very low fat!

Be Careful About Fat

Dr. Whitaker says, "My studies show that if you drink just one glass of cream—or a beverage or food containing this amount of cream—your oxygen supply drops so much you run the risk of an angina attack! If you eat a high-fat breakfast of ham, fried eggs, and buttered toast, the same reaction may occur. In addition to your heart, all of your body tissues may become clogged. Your overall health declines." Dr. Whitaker urges you to reduce fat intake, thereby reducing waste intake. You will be rewarded with cleaner arteries and a healthier life.

Food Supplements Are Inner Cleansing

Dr. Whitaker finds that certain supplements bring on an artery-cleansing reaction. He puts his waste-clogged patients on this supplement-cleansing program:

- *Vitamin C:* 1000 to 2000 milligrams with each meal, or a total of 3000 to 6000 milligrams daily.
- *Vitamin E:* "A natural antioxidant," says Dr. Whitaker, "because it boosts the use of cleansing oxygen, protects against certain cancers, helps delay the aging process. Take 400 units daily in any form, although the dry preparations may be better."
- *Vitamin B-complex:* From 10 to 20 milligrams daily of B_1, B_2, B_6, and niacinamide.
- *Vitamin A:* From 10,000 to 15,000 units daily.
- *Vitamin D:* 400 units daily.

What About Minerals?

"Choose a mineral supplement that supplies zinc, chromium, and selenium along with other trace elements. We suggest you check with your physician, though, before starting any supplement program," advises the doctor.

Nutritional Program Boosts Inner Cleansing

"At the beginning of a 12-day session at our center, blood tests are taken with most folks having cholesterol levels of 250 and over. The results at the end of the sessions are cleansing and remarkable. It's not unusual to see cholesterol levels drop from 250 to 150. This is all a result of the diet and exercise program being followed daily," adds Dr. Whitaker. "I gave up surgery because I feel diet and exercise are the ultimate ways to health. Our center is devoted entirely to this new lifestyle to boost better and 'feel-young-forever' health."

Health Rewards

Dr. Whitaker continues, "With this diet program, most folks can say good-bye to many other low-oxygen symptoms such as fatigue, depression, confusion, lethargy and, in many cases, low sex drive." All this and much, much more in refreshing young health is yours when you follow the program. Cleanse your arteries and you enjoy inner (and outer) rejuvenation![22]

FAT—HOW MUCH IS TOO MUCH?

Fat is the most concentrated source of food energy (calories). Each gram of fat supplies about 9 calories, compared to about 4 calories per gram for protein or carbohydrates and 7 calories per gram for alcohol. In addition to providing energy, fat aids in the absorption of certain vitamins. Some fats provide linoleic acid, essential fatty acid which is needed by everyone in small amounts.

Saturated "Bad" Fats

Saturated fats are found in largest proportions in fats of animal origin. These include fats in whole milk, cream, cheese, butter, meat, and poultry. They are also found in large amounts in some vegetable oils, including coconut and palm oil. If a fat hardens at room temperature, it poses a risk to your arteries.

Polyunsaturated "Good" Fats

Polyunsaturated fats are found in largest proportions in fats of plant origin. These include sunflower, corn, soybean, and safflower oils. They are also found in legumes, vegetables, and fruits to a lesser amount. Some fish are also sources of polyunsaturated fats. Liquid fats at room temperature are preferred for your health.

Monounsaturated "Neutral" Fats

Monounsaturated fats are found in fats of plant origin. The most common examples are olive oil and canola oil. Very modest amounts of these oils are helpful in washing out wastes.

Careful: All fats, no matter what they contain, supply almost the same number of calories! Easy does it!

HOW MUCH FAT DOES YOUR BODY NEED?

How do you count fat? How do you determine if a food has too much fat for you? A rule of thumb is that you lower your fat intake so that the fat accounts for less than 30 percent of total calories.

Find your weight on the following chart and find your daily activity level. Be honest! The number you see is the amount of fat, in grams, you're allowed to have each day. You should not have more than this . . . but you may have less!

How Much Fat Is in the Food You Buy?

Read the label! Take the total grams of fat per serving. Multiply that number by 9. Divide by the total calories per serving. Multiply by 100 and you have the percentage amount of fat in the food.

FAT GUIDE
Fat (grams)

Weight (Pounds)	Inactive	Lightly Active*
100	40	47
120	48	56
140	56	65
160	64	75
180	72	84
200	80	93
220	88	103
240	96	112

*Lightly Active: Usual activity and 20–30 minute brisk walk daily.

How Much Fat Per Day?

You want to figure out exactly how many grams of fat are allowed per day. Here's how:

1. Calculate how many calories you eat per day. For example, it's 2000.
2. Multiply the number of calories by the percentage of fat you'd like to eat. For example, you decide to follow a 30 percent fat program. This means on a 2000 calorie program, you can eat approximately 600 fat calories a day.
3. Each gram of fat has 9 calories. Divide 600 by 9.
4. You have 67 grams of fat as the amount you may consume each day.

LESS FAT! HOW LOW CAN YOU GO?

Most health groups advise getting 30 percent of calories from fat. But this is a compromise between what is ideal and what is realistic. Others suggest that 20 percent is a reasonable goal and would be advantageous for inner cleansing. A food program with 20 to 25 percent of calories from fat will further reduce the risk of certain cancers, heart disease, stroke, and diabetes. There is a sharp drop in breast and colon cancer at 20 percent fat.

The Doctor Prescribes

"If I had to pick a number," says John W. Anderson, M.D., professor of medicine and clinical nutrition at the University of Kentucky, "the ideal I would pick would be less than 25 percent. If someone stays lean and walks three miles a day, they can eat 25 percent of calories from fat, and 6 to 8 percent saturated fat; that is the ideal situation. And I think with intensive instruction you can get under 30 percent."[23]

You Do Not Have to Eat 30 Percent of Calories From Fat

Note carefully: 30 percent is the upper limit! This figure means you should eat *less* than 30 percent, with less than 10 percent saturated fat and less than 300 milligrams of cholesterol daily. With lower fat intake, you have less sludge and a chance for better health.

SIMPLE EXERCISES SCRUB YOUR ARTERIES IN DAYS

Keep yourself physically active. Do mild exercises and you enjoy an artery-scrubbing reaction in a matter of days. Simple movements help oxygenate your body to protect against toxic overload.

Oxygen Lack = Artery Clogging

Biologically, an oxygen deficiency weakens the lining of the artery, making it more vulnerable to clogging. There is a buildup of sediment in the blood. It clings to the wall of the red blood cells, thickening it. This thick wall makes it difficult for oxygen to move from the red blood cells into the tissues. In other words, sediment makes the skin of the red blood cells "tough" and cleansing oxygen cannot pass through to the lining of the artery.

Problem: Red blood cells are the major carriers of oxygen to body tissues. If they cannot release this oxygen, the arterial linings become accumulated with sludge.

Solution: Increase the oxygen content of your blood; boost its oxygen-carrying ability with the use of daily exercise. Body movement distributes oxygen to your tissues which then release more cleansing energy.

How Exercise Boosts Oxygenated Cleansing

Simple body motions boost the oxygen-carrying capacity of your blood-stream instantly. This automatically helps dissolve and wash out sludge that accumulates in and on your arteries. Invigorating oxygen does more than wash out wastes from your arteries; it cleanses wastes from your blood-stream. Your red blood cells become healthier. Their own membranes become healthfully thin and are able to transfer oxygen more speedily. By providing a suitable supply of oxygen to the lining of your arteries, you are able to clean them and make them more resilient. You can have sparkling clean arteries with the use of exercise-prompted oxygen. About 30 to 60 minutes of brisk walking every day helps prompt this form of inner cleansing.

WHY TRIGLYCERIDE CONTROL IS IMPORTANT TO ARTERIAL YOUTHFULNESS

In the first few hours after eating a typical high-fat meal, the amount of fats called triglycerides (along with cholesterol) in the blood rises sharply. The liver, meanwhile, draws on fat stores to produce more triglycerides and cholesterol for its own ends.

Triglycerides are your body's source of energy. But if not used immediately, they are stored in fat tissues. Since oil and water don't mix, your body must immediately wrap the triglycerides-cholesterol packages in a protein that dissolves in water, so they may be carried by the blood. As the fat-protein packets (lipoproteins) are passed along they are broken down into smaller packages and rewrapped in new proteins.

Danger of Triglyceride Overload

One fat-protein is low-density lipoprotein (LDL) which causes heart disease when circulating at high levels. Another, very-low-density lipoprotein (VLDL) is choked with triglyceride, suspected of causing cardiovascular problems. There is also the high-density lipoprotein (HDL) which is believed beneficial since it is a form in which cholesterol is pulled out of tissues and brought to the liver for elimination.

A blood test will tell you the proportions of these fats in your bloodstream. Your health specialist can do this test for you.

Why You May Have Excessive-Triglycerides

Daily, some 70 to 150 grams of these waste-forming substances enter your body because you consume foods from two taboo groups: (1) refined carbohydrates such as sugars and starches, and (2) hard animal-source fats. This causes *hypertriglyceridemia,* a vascular risk problem that clogs your arteries.

Triglyceride blood levels are high if you are overweight. You may be carbohydrate-sensitive: sugars and refined starches and large amounts of alcohol raise your readings. Women who take oral contraceptives may also have raised levels.

What Are Safe Readings?

Normal triglyceride levels are based on age. Up to age 30, normal is less than 140 milligrams of triglyceride per deciliter of blood serum. For people aged 30 to 39 normal is less than 150 milligrams. For people aged 40 to 49, normal is less than 160. In those aged 50 and older, normal is less than 190. CAUTION: At any age, if you have a reading of 200 or over, you are at risk and need to start inner cleansing promptly. In other words, keep it under 200.

FATTY ACID TRANSPORT

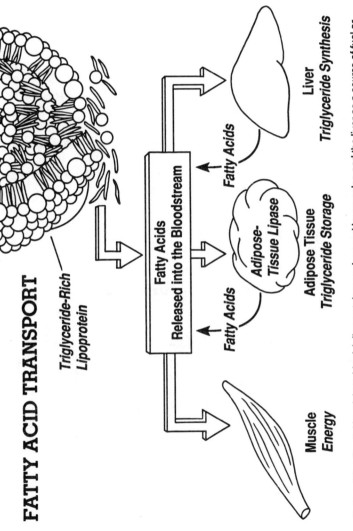

Triglyceride-Rich
Lipoprotein

Fatty Acids
Released into the Bloodstream

Fatty Acids

Fatty Acids

Adipose-
Tissue Lipase

Muscle
Energy

Adipose Tissue
Triglyceride Storage

Liver
Triglyceride Synthesis

Fatty acids released by triglyceride-rich lipoproteins can be used by muscles and the liver as a source of fuel or resynthesized into triglycerides for storage in the liver or adipose-tissue. When too many triglycerides accumulate, they can be released back into circulation in the form of fatty acids where they may line the artery walls, causing atherosclerosis.

Appropriate management of hypertriglyceridemia should be based on several blood tests. Other conditions that are associated with hypertriglyceridemia, such as diabetes and kidney disorders, should be controlled. This assessment should be conducted and evaluated by your health specialist, along with other cardiovascular risk factors that may be present.

SEVEN STEPS TO CONTROL OF "FORGOTTEN" BLOOD FAT

Triglycerides are said to be "forgotten" because they are overshadowed by other blood fats, although they may well be more risky. A seven-step plan for inner cleansing is outlined by Rodolfo Paoletti, M.D., of the Giovanni Lorenzini Medical Foundation, Baylor College of Medicine in Houston, Texas:

1. To bring down blood fats, improve your diet to cut out excessive animal fats and refined sugars and starches.
2. Reduce caloric intake. Less weight—less fat.
3. Lower your weight to an acceptable level.
4. Avoid alcohol.
5. Fat intake should be under 30 percent of total calories.
6. Increase intake of fiber and complex carbohydrates.
7. Daily exercise is essential.

"These basic guidelines will do much to help keep triglyceride and other fat levels at a safer level," says Dr. Paoletti. "Many studies have shown a correlation between elevated serum triglyceride levels and increased risk of coronary artery disease in both men and women. There is increasing evidence that triglycerides contribute to the buildup of plaque in the coronary arteries." He calls for weight reduction and a diet low in saturated fats and cholesterol and rich in complex carbohydrates "as the first steps in treating hypertriglyceridemia, as are exercise and alcohol restriction."[24]

How's Your Reading?

Claude Lenfant, M.D., of the National Heart, Lung, and Blood Institute, Bethesda, Maryland, notes, "Elevated triglyceride levels cannot be dealt with if the treating physician does not know they are present. They have to be measured to evaluate your LDL-cholesterol level. Lipoprotein analysis, including cholesterol, triglycerides, HDL and LDL, provides the physician with valuable information to design a comprehensive treatment program.

"Triglyceride levels should always be tested after an overnight fast and should be measured on two to three separate occasions to eliminate the possibility of laboratory error or a single spurious result." Dr. Lenfant also emphasizes, "Levels over 200 mg/dl deserve attention![25]

Simple Adjustment Controls Problem

Limit or avoid any foods or beverages that contain refined carbohydrates. These are the waste forming sugars and starches that boost triglycerides. Read labels of packaged items. *Tip:* Safer are complex carbohydrates such as whole grain breads and cereals, legumes, and fresh fruits and vegetables.

Control Animal Fat Intake

These boost waste-forming triglycerides. Must have meat? Trim off all visible fat before cooking and then before eating. Switch to less-fatty poultry and fish.
   Vegetable Oils? Use in Moderation
   On the average, one tablespoon of most oils has about 115 calories and about 13.0 grams of fat. And 100 percent of the calories come from this vegetable fat. A small amount of vegetable oil may be used because it has polyunsaturates which help control artery-clogging triglycerides—but easy does it. If you must, use two or three tablespoons as your limit each day.

CASE HISTORY—**Lowers Dangerous Triglycerides in Seven Days**

Constant trembling, nervous upset, fuzzy memory threatened the auditing position of Ronald I. B. He tired easily, even when sitting most of the day. He could scarcely keep his eyes open by midday. Slightly overweight, he looked haggard and much older than his 50 years. A hematologist (blood specialist) diagnosed his problem as high triglycerides. His arteries were being "choked to death." Ronald I. B. was put on a simple program: NO refined carbohydrates. NO animal fats. NO alcohol. More exercise. Within four days, he had a firm grip, was even tempered, and enjoyed a good memory. He was doubly energetic. In seven days, he was alert, agreeable, and gave the impression of being much younger than his formerly "old" 50 years. His triglyceride levels had dropped down to 180 mg/dl. His arteries were cleansed. Life was so very wonderful.

THE ARTERY-CLEANSING POWER OF GARLIC

Several garlic cloves daily create a powerful detoxification reaction within your system. Garlic has a dilating effect on your blood vessels; it scours away wastes and helps balance your blood pressure.

In particular, it is the *allicin* (active sulfur-containing ingredient in garlic) that helps balance the lipid (fat) levels in your bloodstream. Allicin helps break down fatty clumps in your liver and other vital organs, releasing and helping to eliminate them so you have cleaner arteries.

Detoxification Plan

Have several garlic cloves daily. Eat garlic raw (use parsley or a cinnamon stick afterward to avoid becoming a social outcast) and use in cooking, too. (No odor when garlic is cooked.) Garlic helps you clean your arteries . . . while you eat!

THE OMEGA-3 WAY TO CORRECT "METABOLIC SLUGGISHNESS" AND "SMOGGY OXYGEN"

These two problems are the forerunners to plaque or waste buildup. A weak metabolism and a waste-filled oxygen supply give toxins a chance to accumulate. You need to have a more vigorous metabolism and stronger oxygen availability to dislodge wastes. Otherwise, the situation in your body is similar to that of a stagnant pool. It becomes a cesspool of debris and is toxic to anyone who comes in contact with the putrid blockage. There is one way to initiate an internal whirlpool to dislodge and wash out accumulated wastes. Here it is.

Omega-3 Fatty Acids

Certain types of fish contain large amounts of detoxifying fatty acids such as eicosapentaenoic (EPA) and decosahexaenoic (DHA), said to be more effective than polyunsaturated fats in scrubbing away fatty deposits.

Both EPA and DHA fatty acids are also able to lower blood levels of triglycerides and cholesterol; these same detoxifying acids reduce both the numbers and stickiness of clot-forming blood platelets. They may also reduce the formation of artery-clogging fatty plaques on the walls of blood vessels and counter arterial spasms that interfere with blood flow and raise blood pressure.

Omega-3 fatty acids with the detoxifying EPA and DHA have the ability to transfer oxygen from the blood to your muscle tissues. They further influence the release of oxygen in your muscles, too, and speed up your sluggish metabolism. The omega-3 fatty acids prompt internal "air conditioning" so that smoggy body pollutants are "blown away." You are rewarded with a refreshingly good feeling. It is similar to sparkling sunshine after a sudden thunderstorm. Everything becomes fresh and pure and clean. So it is with your body, thanks to the magic of the omega-3 fatty acids.

Omega-3 Detoxifying Program

Potent sources of this cell scrubber include: Atlantic mackerel, pink salmon (canned), Atlantic salmon, Atlantic herring, sablefish, whitefish, chinook salmon, sockeye salmon, bluefin tuna, and coho salmon.

Several times per week, include any of these types of fish on your menu. You will be giving your metabolism the needed omega-3 fatty acids needed to scrub away toxic accumulations from your arteries.

CASE HISTORY—Overcomes Arteriosclerosis, Restores Youth

Told by her internist that she had dangerously high blood fat levels and thick porridge-like clumps of wastes that were choking her arteries, Helga DeH. was eager to correct this life hazard. She followed her internist's guidelines calling for low- or no-animal fat foods. She went for 60-minute walks twice a day. She also boosted her intake of seafood which had the detoxifying omega-3 fatty acids. Within nine days Helga DeH. was diagnosed as having youthful arteries, cleansed of waste. She was the picture of health, too. She felt restoration of youth, thanks to this easy and speedy detoxification plan.

Clean Arteries Today—Youthful Life Tomorrow

Protect your arteries from sludge and enjoy an oxygenated and blood-nourished circulatory system. These detoxification programs work swiftly and effectively. Begin today and experience the joys of youth tomorrow.

------------------------------ *HIGHLIGHTS* ------------------------------

1. *Unclog your arteries, cleanse away sludge to feel better.*
2. *A doctor outlines a detoxification program that lowers excess fat and helps you overcome "aging" arteriosclerosis.*
3. *Simple exercises will scrub your arteries in days.*
4. *Control the "forgotten" fat—triglycerides—for arterial youthfulness. Garlic is one important inner cleaner.*
5. *Ronald I. B. lowered his dangerous triglycerides in seven days.*
6. *Omega-3 fatty acids in seafood help clean away sticky platelets.*
7. *Helga DeH. overcame arteriosclerosis with a simple program within nine days.*

Chapter 14

HOW BODY MOTIONS WASH AWAY STUBBORN ACHES AND PAINS

Wash away accumulated debris clinging to your cells and tissues and ease-erase stubborn aches and pains. Muscle tissue frequently becomes cluttered with metabolic wastes. They cause irritation erupting in backaches, neck pains, leg cramps, and a general feeling of achiness. Blame the hurt on your inactivity. "Rust" (metabolic wastes) clings to your important organs, making it difficult to get around. Only when this rust is washed away, can you become more flexible. Your cells, muscular system, and vital organs can all be at high risk to this congestion. You need to keep them active so that any rust that does accumulate can be shaken loose and washed out of your body, freeing you from hurt.

BODY MOTIONS DETOXIFY YOUR WASTES

Simple body motions or exercise programs help dislodge stubborn clinging wastes and cleanse your various systems and organs so there is less hurtful blockage of your movements. Body motions help free you from these ache-causing wastes. Some detoxification benefits of these easy-to-do body motions are:

- You'll cleanse your blood circulation. Your vital organs and muscles will work more efficiently, without any sediment-causing pains.
- Exercise washes away dirt from your nerve cells. You become stronger when facing the stresses of daily living.
- Simple exercises dislodge toxic wastes from your bones, ligaments, and tendons. Clean organs can function without grating pain.
- Body motions stimulate your cleansed lungs to absorb more oxygen. Your blood is enriched by an increase in oxygen-carrying hemoglobin to nourish your muscles. Cleansed, they contract and expand without painful protest.

Detoxification Boosts Inner Cleansing

Regular exercise at least 30 minutes a day should help you perspire. In so doing, you cleanse your inner organs and are rewarded with these benefits:

- Heavier breathing invigorates the mucosal sheath that coats your respiratory tract and washes out toxins.
- When you perspire, there is an acceleration of oxygen going in and out of your lungs. Perspiration stimulates excretion of toxic wastes through sweat, bile, stool, and urine.
- Within 15 minutes of a sweat-producing exercise session, you experience an invigoration of your adrenal glands. There is an outpouring of epinephrine (adrenalin) and norepinephrine (noradrenalin), hormones that rejuvenate blood circulation and important metabolic-excretion processes.
- Sustained body motions mobilize fat in which toxic chemicals (pesticides, pollutants, poisons) are gathered, uprooting them for elimination.
- Hearty exercise alerts your pituitary gland to release endorphins, morphine-like substances that soothe pain and help you feel glad all over. You are "bathed" in natural pain-killers.

These are bonus benefits as you develop an improved body image and self-awareness. You experience more vitality and joy of living. You will enjoy many rewards as simple body motions uproot and shake loose stubborn "body rust" that causes distressing aches and pains.

EASY BODY MOTIONS CLEANSE BURSITIS TOXEMIA

Bursitis is traced to the accumulation of calcium-like wastes that have accumulated in certain pockets of your body. A *bursa* is a sac situated between two structures, such as between skin and bone, between tendons and bone, and so on. Incompletely metabolized calcium or accumulated toxic wastes gather in the bursa, giving rise to pain.

While you have these bursa pockets in your elbows, hips, and knees, the most common area of distress is around the shoulder. Calcium wastes accumulate in one of the tendons that elevates your arm when you put on your coat, reach into a back pocket, brush your hair, or perform daily chores. There is a sharp pain, caused by the grating irritation of these wastes that block free movement of your arms. To detoxify bursitis toxemia, simple body motions will clean your tendons and provide youthful flexibility.

Horizontal Arm Circles

Stand erect, arms extended sideward at shoulder height, palms up. Make small circles backward with hand and arms. Reverse, turn palms down and do small circles forward. Repeat fifteen to twenty times.

Shrug Away Bursitis Pain

Stand erect, hands at sides. Gently rotate your shoulders up, back, down and around. Repeat ten to fifteen times.

Arm Swing and Flex

Stand erect, arms at sides, hands upward at chest level. Swing both arms together forward and back. On the forward swing, flex both elbows, drawing your fists toward your shoulders. *Note:* Inhale while your arms swing forward and back. Exhale vigorously as you bring them down again. Repeat fifteen times.

Book Holding for Shoulder Freedom

Stand erect, arms extended overhead. Hold a book in each hand. (1) Bend arms at elbows, slowly lowering your book-holding hands. (2) Keep elbows as high as possible, close to your head. (3) Extend arms slowly as you return to starting position. Repeat three sets up to ten times.

Cleanses, Refreshes, Restores Flexibility

These easy body motions are directed at detoxifying the crystal-like wastes that are broken up and excreted from your body. With restored flexibility, you can say goodbye to waste-caused bursitis.

CASE HISTORY—Eight Years of Bursitis Conquered in Eight Days

Ordinary household chores became agony for Adele Y. C. as the years went by. Her shoulder pains became so intense, she would scream and then sob after making an unexpected shoulder twist. She feared her bursitis would make her an invalid. A physiotherapist suggested she detoxify the clogging deposits and cast them out of her bursa pockets. Adele Y. C. followed the prescribed body motions as outlined above. She was amazed. Her flexibility was restored within a few days. At the end of eight days, she was as agile as a youngster. Detoxification conquered her agonizing bursitis problem of eight years in only eight days.

EASY LEG-EXERCISES MELT AWAY TOXEMIA-CAUSED CRAMPS

Those stiff legs that make you pause for breath every few steps are in need of washing—not externally, but internally. The waste accumulations in your legs become locked in joints, ligaments, tendons, cells, even in your bloodstream. Here, they become glue-like, restricting free leg movement. You know it is toxemia when you feel a sharp, stabbing sensation while trying to bend your knees. Often, in the middle of the night, you feel severe leg cramps. You need to uproot and cast out accumulated toxic wastes. Here is a set of fun-to-do body movements. They unlock debris from your hips right down to your toes. Within moments, you feel the heaviness lifting and a more youthful flexibility returning to your legs. Wash out the debris and restore comfort and strength to your legs.

Quick Leg Revitalization Movement

Stand on one foot; hold onto something for balance. Keep your back straight. Using your free hand, pull your knee toward your chest. Don't strain. Get an easy stretch. Gradually, increase the action from 10 to 30 seconds. Repeat three times.

Lower Leg Rejuvenation

Put the ball of your foot on the edge of a curb or stair, with the remaining part of your foot hanging down over the edge. Lower heel down below level of curb where the ball of your foot is resting. Go slowly, working on balance. (You may have to hold onto something for support.) Keep leg on which your Achilles tendon and ankle are being stretched as straight as possible. Be relaxed before increasing the stretch. Work on feeling a good stretch. Slowly does it. Repeat up to five times.

Easy Knee Bend

Stand erect, hands on hips, feet comfortably spaced. Bend knees to 45°, keeping your heels on the floor. Return to starting position. Do it again. Repeat ten to fifteen times and gradually work up to twenty times.

Calf Raise

Stand erect, hands on hips, feet spread 6 to 12 inches apart. Raise your body up on your toes, lifting your heels. Return to starting position. Keep breathing deeply. Repeat up to five sets. This is a simple, yet remarkably exhilarating detoxifying exercise that dislodges and eliminates wastes promptly. It restores youthful flexibility and freedom from pain to your lower limbs.

CASE HISTORY—Frees Legs of Lifetime Pain in Six Days

Nearly crippled by agonizing leg pains, Hugo O'N. had such stiffness he was either confined to a chair or faced the unhappy prospect of having to use a wheelchair. Standing or walking for a short distance brought such cramps, he had to sit down and gasp for breath. Fearing crippling, he sought help from a holistic health practitioner, one who treated the entire body rather than just the symptoms. The practitioner tested Hugo O'N. and diagnosed his problem as toxemia. Sludge deposits were glued together in the cells and tissues of his lower extremities. This toxemia was causing serious blockages. He prescribed the preceding set of leg-ercises. Hugh O'N. followed them. Immediately, he felt the "shackles" removed from his legs. In only six days, he was totally free of the crippling pain. To celebrate, he entered a jogging marathon and finished second! Only 20 to 30 minutes of leg-ercises daily washed away the toxemic blockages and transformed him from an invalid to a champion!

CASTING OUT "STABBING ACHES"

An ache that appears suddenly, then just as suddenly is gone only to have lodged elsewhere in your body, is a much-disliked and feared "stabbing ache."

Why Does It Strike?

Your blood system becomes overburdened with accumulated toxic wastes. As blood flows throughout your body, the sediment spills over and becomes attached to your muscles, tendons, cells, tissues, and bones. These toxic wastes clump together, sometimes for a brief time. A sudden ache is the reaction. Soon, the clump dissolves only to find another gathering site. This is the location of a repeat ache. This "stabbing ache" situation requires simple body motions to stimulate better detoxification of wastes.

How To Strike Back

Carry out as many of the following detoxification motions each day as it is comfortable to do. They will break up toxic clumps and wash them out of your body.

Seated Toe Touch

With toes pointed, as you sit on a carpeted floor, slowly slide hands down legs until you feel a stretch. Hold position and gently try to increase the stretch. Grasp ankles and slowly pull until your head approaches your legs. Relax. Draw your toes back. Slowly try to touch toes. Repeat five times.

Knee Pull

Pull leg to chest as you sit on a carpeted floor, and hold for a count of 5. Repeat with opposite leg (eight to ten times for each leg).

Toe Pull

Seated on the carpeted floor, pull on your toes while pressing legs down with your elbows. Repeat five times.

Wall Stretch

Stand 3 feet from wall, with feet slightly apart. Put both hands on wall. With heels on ground, lean forward slowly and feel stretch in calves. Hold position for 15 to 20 seconds. Repeat five times.

Standing Toe Touch

Stand with legs straight and *slowly* bend over; reach for your toes as far as is comfortably possible. Hold for count of 5. Straighten up. Repeat five times.

Side Bender

Extend one arm overhead, other on hip. Slowly bend to side; hold the stretch and try to reach farther to loosen debris from pockets. Repeat five times for each side.

Jumping Jack

Stand with arms at side. On count 1, jump and spread feet apart, simultaneously swing arms over head. On count 2, return to starting position. Use a rhythmic, moderate cadence. Repeat fifteen to twenty-five times.

When Should You Do These Exercises?

The best time for these motions is either after breakfast or about one hour before your evening meal. Take about 30 minutes to do as many of the preceding body motions as comfortably as possible. They do much to dislodge wastes and prepare them for elimination. Once detoxified, your body is free of debris-causing "stabbing aches."

WASHING THE INSIDES OF YOUR FEET FOR FREEDOM FROM ACHES

You wash the outsides of your feet. Good! Now you need to wash the insides. That is, with the use of simple exercises, you can increase the circulation flowing to your feet and boost detoxification that will do away with recurring aches. Remember, your feet are farthest from your heart; they are usually the first to become sluggish because of waste pileup. With simple foot exercises, you can wash away accumulated debris and become more flexible.

Why Exercises Stimulate Inner Cleansing

If your circulation becomes sluggish, there is a toxic buildup in your cells. Wastes, including lactic acid and other debris, become lodged in your arteries and veins, blocking blood from circulating freely. You develop internal toxemia with distress showing itself as pain. The following set of exercises helps your muscles pump refreshing clean blood back to your heart. The exercises also open your venous valves to stimulate a freer exchange of oxygen and waste, detoxifying your body. Your feet and other limbs become stronger and more flexible. You feel glad (and young) all over. Here goes . . .

1. Sit, relaxed, with bare feet on your carpeted floor or on a towel. Try to pick up a pencil with your toes. *Detoxifying benefit:* Washes wastes from the tendons on top of your feet.

2. Sit in a relaxed position. Cross one leg over the other. Bend your top foot down and then up. Rotate your foot in one direction, then another. Do this up to fifteen times for each foot. *Detoxifying benefit:* Washes wastes from ankle joints to relieve stiffness.

3. Stand on bare feet. Rise up on toes, and then back down again. Repeat ten times. *Detoxifying benefit:* Cleanses debris from your ankles and arches.

4. Stand. Roll your feet outward up to fifteen times until your weight rests comfortably on the outer borders of your feet. *Detoxifying benefit:* Washes away debris from your inner arches to relieve strain.

5. Stand with feet together. Bend toes up as far as you can. Repeat ten times. *Detoxifying benefit:* Cleanses toxic wastes from the muscles of your toes.

6. Stand. Keep both legs straight as you cross them (as a scissors) with feet flat on the floor and slightly apart. Distribute body weight evenly between both feet. Hold this position for the count of 30. Reverse. Repeat. *Detoxifying benefit:* Cleanses impediments from the muscles controlling foot and leg balance.

7. Sit on a carpeted floor with both legs extended straight ahead. Flex your feet back as far as is comfortably possible. Repeat ten times. *Detoxifying benefit:* Washes cells of the calf and heel muscles.

8. Sit on carpeted floor with both legs extended straight ahead. Turn soles of your feet closely together (as if clapping your soles together). Repeat ten times. *Detoxifying benefit:* Cleanses debris from arches and tones up calf muscles through tendon-ligament washing.

9. Lean against wall. Put your weight on your arms. Now, kick yourself gently in the back of your upper thigh with heel of foot. Easy does it. Do this with each foot. *Detoxifying benefit:* Dislodges wastes in your thigh muscles to promote greater flexibility.

10. Lie flat on carpeted floor or on a bed. Bend your knee. (That grating noise is a disloding of nitrogenous wastes.) Grasp your leg with both hands. Gently pull your knee back towards your body. Repeat 5 times. *Detoxifying benefit:* Loosens and washes out deposits and sludge in your knees to give you more flexibility.

Your Personal Schedule

Only 30 minutes daily! That's all you need to promote detoxification-washing of the "insides" of your feet. You will invigorate important metabolic processes to exhilarate your lower limbs and the rest of your body.

———————————— *HIGHLIGHTS* ————————————

1. *Adele Y. C. overcame eight years of bursitis by performing easy body motions for only eight days.*

2. *Melt away toxemia-caused cramps with easy leg-ercises. Hugo O'N. freed his legs of "lifetime" pain in only six days with this simple at-home program.*

3. *Cast out "phantom aches" with easy waste-washing detoxification motions.*

4. *Free your feet from aches with "inside washing" exercises. Only 30 minutes daily boosts total body flexibility.*

Chapter 15

HOW TO DE-AGE YOUR CELLS AND MAKE YOUR BODY BRAND NEW AGAIN

Every part of your body is made of cells. The cleaner your cells, the younger-feeling your body. Since your trillions of cells are involved with your vital functions, you can recognize the importance of using home programs for inner cleansing. With sparkling clean cells, you are rewarded with an equally sparkling and youthfully fresh body and mind.

CLEAN CELLS = TOTAL REJUVENATION

You have cells whose chief task is to metabolize valuable oxygen. You have cells whose main function is to receive and dispatch stimuli. You have cells which work to enable you to contract or expand your muscles. You have cells which release fluids, and cells which transport nutrients from one part of your body to another. Some cells carry iron in hemoglobin to nourish your bloodstream. To perform these endless tasks, your cells must be clean of accumulated wastes. Then they are able to carry out their obligations in keeping your body healthy, repairing your vital organs, building immunity to illness, and helping you look and feel youthfully alert.

Cells Influence Health Levels and Immune Response

Each cell has its own health job to perform. One cannot be substituted for another. One group of cells will absorb food and oxygen; another group will wash out wastes, another group will build your immune system. All this is possible with clean and detoxified cells that determine your level of health.

Looking at Your Cells

To know how to keep your cells clean, let's look at the basics about this smallest unit of your body capable of independent life. A cell is a tiny jelly-like blob. It consists of *cytoplasm,* a protein solution, in a fine but strong container called the *membrane.* Most cells have a dense kernel, the *nucleus,* which influences the activity of the rest of the unit. A cell contains a set of *organelles,* visible only with an electron microscope. These are tiny structures which have enclosing membranes, hardly more than a molecule thick.

Foundation of Your Health

Among the organelles found deep within your cells are *mitochondria.* This is the target zone or bullseye of your health. It is in your mitochondria that nutrient combustion takes place to provide energy and vitality for your cell's activities. This means that sparkling clean mitochondrial structures are able to create this nutrient metabolism. Your cells become superinvigorated, able to perform at top efficiency levels. Your reward is a look and feel of overall youthful vitality. So you can readily appreciate the importance of having clean cells for healtheir mitochondria. Your entire body reacts with energy and stamina.

FREE RADICALS AND PREMATURE AGING

Oxygen, although essential for life, also participates in a series of biological reactions that can damage or even destroy living cells and the tissues and organs that they form. Oxygen-containing free radicals are byproducts of normal body metabolism that can destroy a cell or impair its ability to function. Cell, tissue and organ injury, inflammation, cancer, cardiovascular distress, arthritis, and premature aging have all been tied to an excess of the highly reactive compounds known as free radicals. They can cause severe injury or cellular death and decrease the activity and availability of neurotransmitters (molecules that carry chemical messages between nerve cells). Free radicals can attack many molecules that venture into their vicinity within your body!

Threats to Your Immune System

Your immune system is constantly bombarded by free radicals. They are present in air pollution, tobacco smoke, rancid fats. They are common byproducts of normal metabolism. They assault your immune system around the clock. DANGER: Unchecked, they could cause severe, irreversible damage to tissues. For example, assault on your cell membrane results in reduced capability of that membrane to transport nutrients, oxygen, and water into the cell and to regulate inner cleansing of cellular waste products.

Premature aging, impaired immune function, cancer, atherosclerosis, and many other health complications have been linked to the free radical damage of cells and tissues.

ANTIOXIDANTS SAVE YOUR (YOUTHFUL) LIFE . . . AND THEN SOME

Your body has a remarkable defense against free radical toxemia—a set of antioxidants (natural substances containing certain nutrients) that can prevent or delay the oxygen-caused deterioration of your molecules. These antioxidants act as cell scrubbers; they protect your immune system against the assault of these highly reactive (due to an unpaired electron) and unstable byproducts of oxygen metabolism.

How Your Body Defends Itself

Your body is able to defend itself with antioxidants—nutrients that boost your immune response. These nutrients can prevent damage from oxidation. For example, a peeled apple turns brown because of cell damage caused by free radicals, but it stays white if lemon juice, rich in antioxidants, is squeezed on it. These same nutritional antioxidants can slow the aging process. Why?

In simple language, you don't get old. You "rust" from oxidation—from the free oxygen radicals. Antioxidants can help your body defend itself against this "rust."

What Is an Antioxidant?

An antioxidant is a substance that opposes oxidation or inhibits reactions produced by oxygen or peroxides. An antioxidant has properties that protect the vital fatty acids of your body from destruction. Through inner cleansing, it can keep your nerves and cells healthy and more disease-resistant.

Remember, there is no escaping the health threat of free radicals. You expose your body every minute of the day to deterioration by free radicals because of what you eat, drink, breathe, and do (or don't do). Free radicals cause the cell membranes and fatty acids to oxidize, which in turn weakens your immune system and allows entrance of illness and increased aging. Fight back—with nutritional antioxidants!

NUTRIENTS FOR INNER YOUTH THROUGH CELLULAR CLEANSING

Deepening wrinkles, gray hairs, increasing tiredness . . . more than visible signs of aging. Rather, there is internal damage that has been allowed to accumulate over a lifetime. This aging "may be linked to those mischievous molecules inside us called free radicals," says Sheldon Hendler, M.D., Ph.D., of the University of California at San Diego, [where he practices internal medicine as a professor, too.] "Some nutrients called antioxidants help protect the body from free radical damage, giving them claim to anti-aging effects."

Dr. Hendler has found that these nutritional antioxidants can neutralize free radicals by pairing up their electrons. These antioxidants promote inner cleansing and wash out excessive free radicals, decreasing their threat to your health. These valuable antioxidants include:

Vitamin A. "There are hundreds of papers demonstrating that vitamin A can suppress the malignancy of cultured cells transformed by radiation, chemicals, or viruses, delay the development of transplanted tumors and completely prevent malignancy in subjects exposed to potent carcinogens." This vitamin boosts the immune system and accelerates wound healing. *Food Sources:* sweet potatoes, carrots, cantaloupe, broccoli, peaches, squash, green and yellow fruits, vegetables.

Vitamin C. Dr. Hendler says, "Ascorbic acid is being seriously investigated with results related in particular to immunity and prevention of cancer. There is impressive evidence that vitamin C blocks the cancer-promoting effects of nitrosamines. Disease-fighting white blood cells are partly dependent upon this vitamin for normal functioning. Vitamin C may have mild antiviral effects. High doses boost the production and activity of interferon, a virus-fighting substance produced by the body." *Food Sources:* oranges, grapefruits, green peppers, broccoli, papayas, brussels sprouts, cantaloupe, and citrus fruit juices.

Vitamin E. "Protects against cardiovascular disease and problems of intermittent claudication, a painful narrowing of the leg arteries," says Dr. Hendler. People with this condition who took 300 to 800 international units of vitamin E daily for at least three months had more success in overcoming disorders. It is known that this vitamin does have strong antioxidant properties. *Food Sources:* wheat germ oil, sunflower seeds, raw wheat germ, sunflower seed oil, almonds, pecans, hazelnuts, unrefined cereal products, and many legumes such as soybeans, peas, beans.

Selenium. "There is no dispute over selenium's cancer-fighting, anti-oxidant effects," says Dr. Hendler. In tests, selenium added to drinking water significantly reduced the incidence of liver, skin, breast, and colon cancers. Selenium is a powerful stimulant of the immune system, increasing antibody production. It appears to rejuvenate the heart, making it an important nutrient for immunity against cardiovascular distress. *Food Sources:* seafood, whole grain bread and cereal, broccoli, cabbage, onions. (The amount of selenium in foods varies according to the level of this mineral in the soils where they are produced. In general, soils in the west contain more selenium than those in the east. CAUTION: Excessive amounts of selenium may be toxic; do not go over a dosage of 200 micrograms daily without supervision of your health practitioner.)

Zinc. "Acts as an antioxidant and has been found to be a potent immune system booster," says Dr. Hendler. "Adequate zinc is essential to the development and maintenance of a healthy immune system. Aging associated with immune impairment can sometimes be partially repaired with zinc supplementation." It is also involved in the maintenance of taste, smell, and vision; in wound healing; in maintaining male sex drive and fertility; and as an anti-inflammatory agent. *Food Sources:* brewer's yeast, beans, nuts, seeds, wheat germ, seafood, and liver (but this is also high in fat and cholesterol.)

Dr. Hendler suggests you see your health practitioner about supplements. "People like us have to be the pioneers in this area. Within the next 20 years, authorities will recommend increased antioxidant supplementation."[26]

THE VITAMIN THAT RESTORES "YOUNG POWER" TO YOUR CELLS

Vitamin C is unique in providing your organelles with supercharging energy to invigorate "young power" from head to toe.

Provides Energy, Cellular Rejuvenation, De-aging. Vitamin C prompts your mitochondrial structures to absorb more oxygen. This process improves cellular washing. Rejuvenation occurs when vitamin C detoxifies your aged cells and replaces them with new ones. Vitamin C rejuvenates your *osteoblasts* (bone-forming cells). It repairs the fibrous or tissue parts of your body. Without vitamin C, the osteoblasts and fibroblasts (tissue makers) are weakened, even halted. This could bring on aging. You need vitamin C available at all times in adequate amounts to protect against cellular toxemia.

VITAMIN C REBUILDS "AGING" SKIN CELLS

Once vitamin C enters your bloodstream, it speedily prepares *collagen,* an abundant protein needed to detoxify and repair your aging tissues. Fibrous, tough, and pliant, collagen (its name is derived from the Greek word for glue) is needed to rebuild your skin, cartilage, bone, tendons, ligaments, arterial walls, nerve sheaths, and vital organs. Collagen needs vitamin C for its own manufacture; then collagen is able to repair and regenerate your aging cells. But even more important, vitamin C scours, cleanses, and washes your mitochondria. This inner cleansing helps de-age your cells and rejuvenate your body.

How Vitamin C Rejuvenates Your Skin

When assimilated by your digestive system, vitamin C is oxygen-transported via your bloodstream to your cells. The vitamin speedily promotes the mitochondria cleansing; then it is used to perk up aged skin. Vitamin C is absorbed by your body's inner cells and blood vessels. Soon, it becomes a living part of your skin tissue. But before this can be done, your cells need to be cleansed so vitamin C can be absorbed through the cell membrane and enter its nucleus. Once this is accomplished, your skin undergoes a transformation. It becomes firm, smooth, and young again. Rebuilding and rejuvenating your skin is an "inside" job, thanks to the work of vitamin C.

Citrus Juices Detoxify-Rebuild Cells

A powerful concentration of vitamin C is found in fresh citrus juices. These are grapefruits, oranges, tangerines, lemons, and limes. Freshly squeezed citrus juice is a prime source of enzymes, too. These are protein-like miracle workers that energize vitamin C and prompt it to perform its detoxifying-rebuilding of your cells. A few glasses of fresh citrus juice daily influences the health of your mitochondria and boost the manufacture of cell-rejuvenating collagen.

"Wonder Youth Tonic"

To prepare, squeeze, blenderize, or extract the juice from any citrus fruit. Try a combination of fruits with a squeeze of lemon or lime. Add a half teaspoon of honey for added flavor. *Special Boost:* Crush a 1000-milligram tablet of vitamin C (from any health store) into the tonic for super-power. Drink one glass after breakfast, another after your noon meal, and a third at the end of your evening meal.

Restores Tissue Integrity, Detoxifies, Cleanses, Refreshes

Enzymes in the raw juice will dispatch the highly concentrated vitamin C through your bloodstream to your trillions of cells. Here, the vitamin works swiftly to reuild your cytoplasm, membranes, mitochondria, osteoblasts, and fibroblasts. At the same time, enzymes plus C will detoxify the accumulated wastes that block nutrient absorption. It is this double cleansing action of (1) restoration and (2) inner scouring that exerts an overall refreshing regeneration of your body and mind. This is the power of the "Wonder Youth Tonic," especially when fortified with a vitamin C tablet for super-cleansing, super-regeneration, and super-detoxification.

More Sources of Cell-Cleansing Vitamin C

This cleansing-regenerating vitamin is found in strawberries, papaya, cantaloupe, tomato, broccoli, green pepper, raw leafy greens, and white and sweet potatoes.

Plan to have a fresh fruit or raw vegetable salad each day. You will be introducing a high concentration of cell-cleansing and cell-rejuvenating vitamin C. This works around the clock in your de-aging process. You will need to cook the potatoes, and some vitamin C will be evaporated, but they are part of a good foundation for cellular cleansing.

CASE HISTORY—Wonder Youth Tonic Detoxifies Body in Three Days

Christopher T. R. began to develop one ailment after another. Blotches cropped up all over his body. Digestive upsets made him skip meals, and become malnourished. His nerves were sensitive. He would snap upon the slightest provocation. His vision was blurred; he caught one cold after another. He walked like a very old man with a "hunched" look because of his rounded shoulders. He showed all the signs of rapid aging, even though he was still in his early fifties. A local cytologist (specialist in cellular rebuilding) diagnosed his problem: waste-laden cells that were starving because of toxic blockages. A simple program was prescribed: more fresh fruits and vegetables. Three times daily, he was to have a glass of "Wonder Youth Tonic." Almost at once, Christopher T. R. responded. His skin cleared, tightened, and became bright again. His digestion was good; he was cheerful again and his eyesight sharpened. He overcame the sniffles. His posture improved. The "hump" straightened. At the end of three days, he felt as if twenty years had been taken off his life. All this because of the raw food program and the powerful detoxifying nutrients in the tonic.

WHY ANIMAL FATS ARE HARMFUL TO YOUR CELLS

An excessive amount of animal fat can be cell-destroying. Free radicals feed on fats!! The problem is that hard fats deposit thick sludge on your mitochondria. Your cells are unable to receive enough oxygen to metabolize foodstuffs completely into energy-producing carbon dioxide and water. Your waste-covered cells become "choked" and die soon. This starts the premature aging syndrome. Normal enzyme activity is altered. Cellular deterioration worsens.

Simple Change Reverses Aging Process

Limit intake of animal foods. Instead of butter, use vegetable oils in moderation. Switch to low-fat or non-fat dairy products. Avoid skin on poultry. Boost intake of fish. These simple changes will spare your cells the waste-forming fats that block free oxygen transfer. You will then help your body reverse the cellular aging process; you will cleanse your mitochondria and open the way to youth restoration.

CASE HISTORY—Says "No" to Hard Fats, Says "Yes" to Eternal Youth

Irked by being called "old man" in his office, Martin Z. took a close look at himself. He ruefully (and silently) admitted he did look aged with his pale skin, sagging chin, blotchy eyes, and general shuffling malaise. He took his problems to an internist who also believed in detoxification as part of total body healing. An exam and blood test showed that Martin Z. had "cellular clogging" because of hard fatty wastes gluing his mitochondria together, like a clogged up sieve. It blocked free transport of oxygen and nutrition. Cellular destruction was diagnosed as the cause of his aging. The internist put him on a detoxification program of no animal fats at all. He could enjoy some fish because it was a source of omega-3 fatty acids and valuable polyunsaturates. He used some vegetable oils in moderation. (No tropical oils from the coconut or palm source because these are higher in saturated fats than most oils.) Martin Z. followed this detoxification program. In four days, he had a firm, youthful skin with no more sag, no blotches, no exhaustion. He had such vitality, he was called "wonder boy" instead of "old man." The easy detoxification program had corrected his cellular deterioration, cleansed his body, and given him the look and feel of eternal youth.

HOW FISH OILS DE-AGE YOUR CELLS AND ADD YOUTHFUL YEARS TO YOUR LIFE

Fish oils help in cellular cleansing. They are a prime source of the valuable omega-3 fatty acids which help scour your cells and remove excessive sludge. Fish should be used regularly; it is also a prime source of vitamin D, the "sunshine vitamin."

Fish Oils Revitalize Lymphatic System

The omega-3 fatty acids bathe your body cells to invigorate antibodies and detoxify white blood cells. Your lymphatic system controls the levels of body wastes. It provides three powerful detoxifying actions which require the omega-3 fatty acids plus vitamin D from fish oils to function. These include:

1. *Blood Protein Cleansing.* The lymphatic system cleanses protein and then deposits it into your blood. You need clean protein to enjoy a youthful bloodstream; it is the omega-3 and vitamin D-energized lymphatics that bring about this detoxification.

2. *Cleans Between Cellular Spaces.* Energized by the omega-3 fatty acids and vitamin D, lymphatics clean spaces between your cells and eliminate toxic wastes such as bacteria, viruses, and infectious substances. *Note:* Your lymphatics cleanse the fluid used to bathe every body cell.

3. *Boosts Resistance to Infection.* Remember, a virus is a germ that causes infections. To build greater immunity, you need to energize your lymphatic system to stimulate your white cells (lymphocytes) to circulate and destroy foreign bodies such as bacteria, parasites, and viruses. This is possible with omega-3 fatty acids and vitamin D.

Energize Your Lymphatic System for Total Detoxification

This detoxifying, waste-washing, virus-fighting system consists of a series of gland-like stations throughout your body. Sometimes called lymph nodes or glands, they are bean-shaped complexes found in your neck, armpits, behind your knees, groin and close to the arteries surrounding your heart. All are connected by a network of slender-walled channels which crisscross your entire body, especially near your arteries and veins. Flowing through this system is the fluid *lymph.* Colorless, it transports nutrients that protect against cellular aging. But your lymphatic system can become waste-burdened and sluggish.

Wastes Block Free Flow of Cleansing Lymph

A backup of wastes slows down lymph flow. The toxic condition is known as *lymphstasis*. Compare it to a clogged kitchen sink drain. If you let the water run, the sink overflows and spills onto the floor.

The same problem happens inside your body during lymphstasis. Accumulating fluid fills up spaces between your cells and cannot be carried off by the lymphatics. *Problem:* A subsequent pileup of fluid and pressure in the intercellular spaces. *Reactions:* Lymph channels in your lungs become so engorged with fluid wastes, they start to stiffen. So will the vital left heart ventricle, which dispatches oxygen-carrying blood throughout your body. This may cause congestive heart failure because of *edema* (fluid buildup).

So you realize that accumulated wastes and liquids cause lymphstasis (stagnation), swelling, and the risk of body breakdown. Wastes become dangerous blockages and threaten your immune system.

HOW FISH OILS IMPROVE LYMPH FLOW

As rich concentrates of omega-3 fatty acids, polyunsaturates, and vitamin D enter your system through fish oils, your lymphatic system becomes alerted. The fish oils stimulate the lymphocytes to release such inner cleansers as macrophages (waste-washers) which devour the toxins and speed their elimination. Fish oils boost the supply of waste-washing lymphocytes and accelerate the power of antibodies (debris-cleansing gamma globulins) and powerful cleansers such as interferon.

Interferon as Natural Cell Washer

Omega-3 fatty acids and vitamin D stimulate the lymphocytes to release the powerful cell cleanser interferon. This dynamic virus fighter scours your cells and works with the macrophages to wash away wastes.

Simple Way to Boost Lymphatic Cleansing Powers

Mix three tablespoons of fish liver oil (available at pharmacies or health stores) in a glass of fresh vegetable juice. Blenderize or stir vigorously. Drink one glass daily. The enzymes in the juice will dispatch the omega-3 fatty acids and vitamin D into your metabolic system within moments after swallowing. Your lymphatic system becomes super-energized, releasing the detoxifying substances. With cleansed cells, you boost your immune system to resist aging. In a short time, you can give yourself a brand-new body, thanks to brand-new cells.

CASE HISTORY—**Conquers Lifetime Disabilities in Twelve Days**

Years of crippling allergies and a depressed immune system weakened Jennifer J. and left her vulnerable to respiratory ailments. She was often confined to a chair. Slight exertion made her gasp for breath and she would have to lie down. Unhappily, she resorted to a wheelchair for longer distances. Saddened by the fear of becoming an invalid, she sought help from a specialist in detoxification. Tests showed she had a serious decline in adequate lymphocytes. Clogged cells locked out the free transfer of important nutrients. Jennifer J. was put on a simple immune boosting program: Eliminate all hard animal fats. Take two tablespoons of fish oil daily. She also had to drink fresh juices daily. Results? Within six days, she could walk unaided. She could breathe deeply. Within ten days, Jennifer J. felt as vigorous as a youngster. She discarded her wheelchair. With her doctor's guidance, she started a fitness program. By the twelfth day, she was pronounced out of the detoxification danger zone. Her "hopeless" disabilities cleared up through detoxification on this nutritional program.

REBUILD LYMPHATIC SYSTEM, REGENERATE CELLS, REJUVENATE BODY, RESTORE POWERFUL IMMUNITY

With the use of improved nutrition, antioxidant nutrients, and fish oils, you are able to exhilarate your lymphatic system to release scouring agents that clean and detoxify your cells. By boosting your immune system, by rejuvenating your virus-fighting and germ-destroying powers, you will have clean cells—your key to a youthful body.

Every living thing consists of cells. They are the controlling forces of your health. Keep them clean and nourished, keep them detoxified and they will keep you more than just healthy—they will keep you invigoratingly youthful. Remember—what is good for your cells is good for every part of you!

——————————— *HIGHLIGHTS* ———————————

1. *Clean up your cells, boost your immune system, and enjoy total rejuvenation with the outlined programs.*
2. *Free radicals can be overcome by antioxidants found in certain foods to save your (youthful) life, says a leading specialist.*

3. *De-age your cells with the cleansing power of vitamin C.*

4. *The tasty "Wonder Youth Tonic" detoxified Christopher T. R.'s body in three days.*

5. *Martin Z. firmed up his body and corrected premature aging with a simple program that eliminated excessive hard fats.*

6. *Detoxifying nutrients in fish oils stimulate your cleansing lymphatic system to build a stronger immune system to fight infections.*

7. *Jennifer J. overcame lifetime disabilities in twelve days through cellular cleansing by boosting her lymphatic system with improved nutrition.*

Chapter 16

FIBER FOR TOTAL CLEANSING

Fiber (or "roughage" as our grandparents called it) is a dynamic cleanser that gives you the feeling of good health within a few hours after consumed. Basically, fiber is the carbohydrate in your diet that cannot be digested. Because of this trait, it is useful in sweeping away debris and helping in its removal. Fiber helps detoxify your body to protect you against hazards of waste overload. This cleansing power makes fiber a valuable substance in terms of internal rejuvenation. It works speedily, effectively, and with little effort on your part. It keeps you younger . . . longer.

MEET THIS DYNAMIC CLEANSER

What Is Dietary Fiber?

This term is given to the components of a food that are not fully broken down in your digestive tract; instead, after it is eaten, it creates a sweeping-cleansing action as it passes through your body and is eliminated. There are two different kinds of fiber.

1. *Insoluble fiber* does not dissolve but provides bulk and helps in the movement of food and water through your intestine. It is best known for promoting regularity. It protects and helps in the treatment of disorders of the intestinal tract like constipation, diverticulosis, hemorrhoids, and cancer of the colon and rectum. *Sources:* whole grains, bran from wheat and corn, whole grain breakfast cereals, some fruits and vegetables.

2. *Soluble fiber* does dissolve in the system and has been found to help lower blood cholesterol levels. It detoxifies your body of bile acids, substances synthesized from cholesterol, prompting your liver to make new bile acids from cholesterol. This process lowers levels of low-density (bad) cholesterol. It also helps diabetes control by slowing absorption of glucose. It controls your appetite by giving you a feeling of fullness or satiety. *Source:* oats, legumes (dried beans, peas, lentils),

guar gum, barley, psyllium seeds, grapefruit, and apple. These two fruits contain pectin, which is beneficial in lowering harmful blood fats.

Foods may contain both insoluble and soluble fibers; some contain more of one type than the other. Many whole grain cereals and breads provide significant amounts of both types of fiber. Fruits, vegetables, and legumes often have a combination of both fibers in varying concentrations; both types are equally important for the role they play in your body's absorption of nutrients. Both work to detoxify your body of wastes.

What Does Fiber Consist of?

Fiber isn't only "roughage." In fact, fiber isn't one substance but a combination of many substances. Basically, fiber consists of cellulose, pectin, hemicellulose, lignin, and gums/mucilages. Found largely in the cell walls of plant foods, these substances are nondigestible in the sense that they do not remain in your body. Instead, they cause an internal sweeping action as they scrub their way through to elimination. For super inner cleansing, you should eat both types. Since different fibers have different detoxifying benefits, you should cover all bases by eating a mix of foods.

FIBER: HOW IT DIGESTS, CLEANSES, HEALS

Fiber is also known as "bulk" or "roughage," although it is not really rough. It does have a sweeping action in your digestive-intestinal system. It also does provide needed bulk. When you eat this magic product, it enters your digestive system where it absorbs available liquid. (It's important to have adequate liquid available when consuming fiber foods.)

Fiber has a water-holding capacity that makes it an effective cleanser. It moves through your intestines somewhat like a sponge, correcting and cleansing metabolism in the *cecum* (pouch in which the large intestine begins). Here it remains for a brief time until ready for elimination, at which time the wastes, toxic debris and pollutants it has picked up along the way are passed out as well.

This internal cleansing initiates effective healing by scrubbing away infectious debris from your vital organs.

Cleanses, Detoxifies Gastrointestinal Tract

When you ingest fiber, you initiate this important two-step cleansing reaction:

1. Fiber prevents waste-forming constipation by decreasing the transit time of food through your intestines. That is, fiber helps expel toxic wastes with less delay. This protects against internal toxemia.

2. Fiber eases straining at the stool. This protects against ailments such as diverticular disease of the colon, irritable bowel syndrome, hemorrhoids, varicose veins, appendicitis, deep vein thrombosis and hiatal hernia. With fiber, the cleansing away of wastes occurs in a short space of time. This reduces pressure and straining and minimizes toxic accumulation; a cleansed gastrointestinal tract rewards you with youthfully good health.

DECREASED TRANSIT TIME IS SECRET OF FIBER'S MAGIC

This unique ability to create bulk and decrease transit time of wastes and debris from storage to elimination makes fiber a dynamic cleansing food. This is the secret of its magic power in stimulating internal cleansing.

Dynamic Detoxification Action

Since fiber holds water, roughage produced by a high-fiber diet is bulkier and softer. The stool passes through the intestines more quickly and easily. This, in turn, means less strain and pressure on your bowels and blood vessels.

As wastes move quickly through the intestines, surrounding tissues are spared excessive exposure to toxins. This decreased transit time protects your internal organs from abuse by toxins. This dynamic cleansing action makes fiber unique in its healing powers.

Fiber Helps Balance Cholesterol Levels

An unusual power of fiber is in its ability to *decrease* the reabsorption of bile salts. These are substances needed to digest and emulsify fats and oils which then become absorbed through the intestines. But if you reabsorb too many bile salts, you risk cholesterol overload.

Fiber compounds "bind" the bile acids, reducing or preventing the reabsorption of bile acid. Reaction? Your body is then "ordered" to draw on its cholesterol stores to synthesize more bile acid. This helps lower your blood (serum) cholesterol levels. Since excess cholesterol may be labelled as waste, it is important to use fiber to sweep it out and maintain healthier levels. For example, it is believed that the soluble fiber beta-glucan found in oat bran helps reduce cholesterol levels when added to a fat-modified diet. It is, indeed, a miracle food!

CASE HISTORY—Controls Cholesterol, Cleanses Bloodstream on Fiber Program

His dangerously high cholesterol readings urged Nicholas U. to seek help from a nutritionist. He was told he had excessive blood sludge in need of speedy cleansing. He needed to reduce his blood cholesterol level, another symptom of excessive toxemia. Nicholas U. was put on a low animal fat program. But more important was boosting intake of fiber. Daily, Nicholas U. was to enjoy a plate of fresh raw vegetables with two tablespoons of cooked beans as well as one tablespoon of bran (from any health store). He had an ample supply of fresh fruits along with legumes and whole grain foods. Within six days, his cholesterol dropped to a safer level. Within nine days, not only did he have a better cholesterol reading, [under 240 mg/dl.], but tests from the nutritionist showed a sparkling clean bloodstream. The fiber had swept away cholesterol wastes and blood sediment. In nine days, he was refreshingly clean and youthful again.

EVERYDAY FOOD SOURCES OF CLEANSING FIBER

The use of fresh, raw, and unprocessed foods is essential for boosting the benefits of cleansing fiber.

Raw vs. Refined

Emphasize more raw foods which provide the desirable bulkier stools, decreased transit time, and lower intro-colonic pressures than refined or processed foods. Refined, processed foods offer minimal amounts of essential roughage. Here is a thumbnail grouping of good dietary fiber foods:

1. *Whole Grains.* These are products that contain the entire grain, that is, the bran or outer layer, the endosperm or starchy middle layers, the germ or fatty inner portion, the grain kernel.
2. *Vegetables.* Raw vegetables are preferred. If cooked, do so just enough to make them palatable. *Tip:* Those vegetables that are chewy or crunchy when raw or slightly cooked are high in cleansing fiber.
3. *Tuberous Root Vegetables.* Carrots, parsnips, white and sweet potatoes, turnips, kohlrabi. *Tip:* The skin is high in fiber, so try to retain this. Even if you must peel them, the vegetables are still excellent sources of detoxifying fiber.

4. *Fruits With Edible Seeds and Vegetables With Tough Skins.* If they contain edible seeds, they are very high in fiber. California dried figs are excellent for fiber and should be eaten regularly. Also include varieties of berries, tomatoes, squash, eggplant.

5. *Pod Vegetables and Legumes.* Eat plenty of green beans, green peas, dried beans and peas, lentils, lima beans.

6. *Seeds and Nuts.* Be sure to chew seeds and nuts very thoroughly. Eat in moderation since they are also concentrated sources of fat.

High Fiber Fruit—California Figs

Dried figs, one of the most ancient of fruits, are one of the very best sources of natural fiber. Those delectable, succulent nuggets, rich in vitamins and minerals and delightful to the taste, are at least 35 percent higher in fiber than 40 percent bran flakes. California dried figs contain more fiber than any other fruit. In approximately 3-1/2 ounces (100) grams of fig (all of it is edible, unlike many other foods), you have nearly 5 grams of fiber. Eating California dried figs, at mealtime or as a quick picker-upper snack, assures that you are adding a source of fiber and good nutrition, not just fillers or empty calories as found in many processed foods.

HOW MUCH FIBER DO YOU NEED EACH DAY?

There are no official recommended daily allowances for fiber, but health authorities have said that about 35 grams of fiber per day helps protect against cancer as well as cholesterol overload; it is also a safe threshold to establish regularity along with daily detoxification. The larger you are in size, the more you need. Thus a small person might require only about 25 grams daily.

As you add more fiber to your diet, drink several glasses of water a day. This helps compensate for any water loss due to the bulking properties of fiber. *Reason:* large amounts of insoluble fibers increase bulk and draw water into the large intestine. The result is a larger, softer stool that exerts less pressure on the colon walls and is eliminated more quickly. Indeed, the reduced pressure also helps prevent diverticulosis (small herniations in the colon wall that may become inflamed).

Fiber + Water Protect Against Cancer

In addition, large amounts of insoluble fibers with water dilute the concentration of potential carcinogens that may be present in the stool. The decreased transit time reduces the exposure of the intestinal wall to those substances. Furthermore, insoluble fiber alters the pH (acid-alkaline balance) of the large intestine, participating in the microbial activity that protects against production of carcinogens. The combined effect may be a reduced risk of colon cancer.

Aim for about 35 grams of fiber daily to detoxify your body and build immunity to many common and uncommon disorders.

THE SINGLE MOST CONCENTRATED SOURCE OF CLEANSING FIBER

In a word, it's *bran,* the outer husk of grains. Bran comes from wheat, corn, rye, oat, rice, or other grain. This outer husk is a rich concentration of valuable detoxifying fiber.

Pure bran passes down into your lower bowel, absorbs water, adds bulk, then promotes a scouring-cleansing-detoxifying action throughout this entire region.

Unique Detoxifying Reaction

Bran prompts an acceleration of waste removal so there is a reduced risk of bacterial infection. Otherwise, loitering microbes can cause deterioration of the gastrointestinal cells and predispose to life-threatening ailments. Bran propels and then discharges these wastes so there is a reduced risk of infestation.

How Much Fiber in Bran?

In only 3-1/2 ounces, you have over 9 grams of fiber. Since one ounce equals 2 tablespoons, you make a simple calculation. Just 7 tablespoons of bran will give you at least 9 grams of this valuable scouring substance.

Ten Cents a Day Keeps Body Youthfully Clean

Keep a "bran shaker" on your table. Throughout the day, sprinkle it over foods. Mix it with juice or soups, on salads; use it in baking bread. Add some to yogurt, flavored with a bit of honey and fresh fruit. Add bran to stews, casseroles, baked goods.

The low cost means that for about ten cents a day you can keep your body youthfully clean and healthy. And bran has a delicious nut-like taste that makes humble food seem extra-special. You can actually eat your way to super health with bran.

FIBER IN SELECTED FOODS

Here is the fiber content of one serving (3½-ounces) of some fruits, berries and vegetables, nuts and seeds. We list only those which have a fiber content of one gram or more.

Food	Grams of fiber	Food	Grams of fiber
Almonds	2.6	Loganberries	3.0
Apples (not pared)	1.0	Macadamia nuts	2.5
Apricots (dried, uncooked)	3.8	Mustard greens (cooked)	1.0
Artichokes	2.4	Okra	1.0
Avocados	1.6	Olives	1.3
Beans, baked	1.5	Parsnips (cooked)	2.0
Beans, lima	1.8	Peanuts (with skins)	2.4
Beans, snap	1.0	Pears (including skin)	1.4
Beechnuts	3.7	Peas, snow	1.2
Beet greens (cooked)	1.1	Peas, cooked	2.0
Blackberries	4.1	Pecans	2.3
Blueberries	1.5	Peppers, raw	1.8
Brazil nuts	3.1	Popcorn	2.2
Broccoli	1.5	Prunes	2.2
Brussels sprouts	1.6	Raspberries	5.1
Cabbage, red	1.0	Rice bran	11.5
Carrots	1.0	Rice polish	2.4
Cashew nuts	2.6	Safflower seed meal	7.4
Celery	1.0	Seaweeds, dulse	3.2
Coconut meat	4.0	Irish moss	1.8
Collard greens	1.2	kelp	6.8
Cowpeas	1.8	laver	3.5
Cranberries	1.4	Sesame seeds, whole	6.3
Cress, garden	1.1	hull removed	2.4
Dandelion greens	1.6	Soybeans, cooked	1.6
Dates	2.3	natto	3.2
Figs (dried)	5.6	miso	2.3
Filberts	3.0	Squash, winter	1.8
Gooseberries	1.9	Strawberries	1.3
Guavas	5.6	Sunflower seeds	3.8
Kale	1.1	Walnuts, black	1.7
Lambs quarters (cooked)	1.8	English	2.1
Lentils	1.2		

CASE HISTORY—**Enjoys Regularity, Digestive Healing, Body Rejuvenation**

Troubled by colitis, unable to eat many foods, and suffering recurring stomach pains, Oliver E. K. sought help from his gastroenterologist. His problem was diagnosed as waste overload as well as irritating debris. Body pollution was "eating away" at his delicate cellular membranes and tissue walls. His physician put him on an easy high-fiber food program. He was also to have about 5 to 7 tablespoons of bran daily added to salads, juices, soups, and baked goods.

Immediately, Oliver E. K. felt relief. Not only did he experience cleansing regularity, but his pains faded away. He was more alert in body and mind. Within six days, he felt totally rejuvenated, thanks to the scouring-cleansing power of simple bran. It added a new taste to foods, too. He no longer had difficulties with his favorite items, either.

Easy Does It

Increasing fiber intake should be gradual, so that digestive discomfort or cramps do not develop. Go slow. And, of course, be sure to drink lots of liquids throughout the day so the fiber can move along comfortably.

"Morning Bran Tonic"

In a glass of fresh vegetable juice, add two teaspoons of unprocessed bran. Add a squeeze of lemon or lime juice for a piquant flavor. Blenderize for 20 seconds. Drink slowly right after your breakfast.

The bran fiber is propelled by the juice enzymes to scour and cleanse your digestive system in the morning. Your cells are washed. They are regenerated through the collagen-forming action of vitamin C from the juice (and from other fruits you eat). You undergo an inner cleansing and cellular detoxification that will make you feel younger than young!

CASE HISTORY—**From Slow Start to Top Speed in Three Days**

Repeated errors at her supervisory job threatened Joan McC.'s position. Her thinking was fuzzy; her speech was slurred; her movements were clumsy—first thing in the morning. This "slow start" extended almost till midday. An efficiency expert suggested she boost her metabolism and detoxify the blockages responsible for her sluggishness. Boosting her intake of fiber foods would help. Also she prepared the "Morning Bran Tonic" each morning. Doing so, Joan McC. felt a revitalization almost from the start. Within three days, she was alert in body and mind. She worked so efficiently, she was recommended for a promotion. A fiber program together with the "Morning Bran Tonic" scoured her internal organs, helped detoxify her cells and tissues, and rejuvenated her metabolism. She was reborn, thanks to this ten-cent-per-portion "magic food."

DISCOVER WHEAT GERM: CELL CLEANSER SUPREME

Wheat germ is part of the seed of the wheat, rich in vitamins, minerals, protein, and cell-cleansing fiber. In 3-1/2 ounces (7 tablespoons), you have close to 3 grams of potent fiber, along with other cell-repairing nutrients.

Double-Action Detoxifying Power

Wheat germ contains octacosanol, a highly potent ingredient that works with fiber to cleanse excess cholesterol, decrease transit time for waste removal, oxygenate your system, and stimulate cellular repair so that you enjoy more vigor, stamina, and endurance. Octacosanol joins with fiber to detoxify your tissues, then initiates the transfer of oxygen from your blood to those cleansed cells. A feeling of detoxification!

Plan to use wheat germ regularly to give yourself the important fiber needed to repair your cleansed cells and make you feel new again.

How to Use Bran or Wheat Germ for Daily Cell Cleansing

Here is a variety of ways to boost fiber intake with the use of both bran and wheat germ. Again, the cost is about ten cents a day. The convenience is obvious. The results will be felt right away.

- Prepare a mixture of wheat germ and bran in skim milk; add sesame seeds and sun-dried fruits with some sliced California figs.
- Stir one teaspoon of bran into your scrambled or poached egg whites.
- Add bran, or wheat germ, or both to your pancake or waffle batter.
- Use a sprinkle of bran instead of croutons as part of a salad or soup.
- Add bran or wheat germ to baked meat, fish, or vegetable loaves.
- Substitute bran or wheat germ whenever a recipe calls for crackers or bread crumbs.
- Add bran or wheat germ to a portion of low- or no-fat cottage cheese and sliced fresh fruits or vegetables for a meal in a cup.
- When baking bread cakes, include wheat germ and bran. For each cup of flour, use up to two tablespoons of either grain. That is, put two tablespoons in your measuring cup, then add your whole grain flour. The taste will be superb, the detoxification enhanced.

When you think of fiber, think of bran and wheat germ. These super foods perform total detoxification of your body. Include other fiber foods and be rewarded with a brand new body . . . from the inside to the outside. For less than ten cents a day, this is your reward. Fiber is your pot of gold at the end of the rainbow of youth.

LEGUMES: THE LITTLE-KNOWN SOURCE OF SUPER-FIBER

Besides being a virtually fat-free, fiber-packed food, beans boast healthy doses of anemia-fighting iron, nerve-soothing B-complex vitamins, and bone-building calcium and phosphorus. Low in sodium and rich in potassium, beans are ideal for anyone with high blood pressure. Because of their amino acids, which combine with other nutrients to form complete protein, beans make an ideal meat substitute.

Legumes include a broad family of beans—kidney, pinto, black-eyed peas, soybeans, chickpeas, lima, navy, lentils—almost all beans are excellent sources of fiber.

For example, 1/2 cup of most beans will give you from 7 to 9 grams of fiber. Legumes offer a change of pace from bran or wheat germ.

Beans, Metabolism, Inner Cleansing

James W. Anderson, M.D., of the University of Kentucky College of Medicine explains that beans and other legumes contain a water-soluble fiber called *pectin* that surrounds wastes and speeds them out of the body before they can cause trouble. In some reported cases, Dr. Anderson tells of men who ate 1-1/2 cups of cooked beans a day and lowered their cholesterol by a whopping 20 percent in only three weeks. "Most people would do well to add about 6 grams of soluble fiber to their diet each day. One cup of cooked beans fits that plan nicely. You're not likely to become bored because you have a variety: navy beans, kidney beans, pinto beans, lima beans, soybeans, black-eyed peas, lentils, etc., all have this cholesterol-lowering ability."

Protects Against Diabetes

When placed on a diet high in fiber-rich beans but very low in fat and sugar, Dr. Anderson found diabetics could greatly improve control of their blood sugar. He tells that many of his patients were able to stop using drugs, including insulin "or significantly reduce the dosage of such drugs. Pectin and gums have the most striking immediate effect on blood sugar, whereas wheat bran (cellulose) seems to offer some long-term benefits." He emphasizes that diabetics should follow this bean fiber program under medical supervision. "I also get nearly a 60 percent reduction in triglyceride levels in those with abnormally high readings by putting them on a high-carbohydrate bean, low-fat diet rich in soluble fibers."[27]

Canned Beans Will Do

While some nutrients are lost during processing, canned beans may be used. To remove any excess salt added during canning, place canned legumes in a strainer. Rinse with cool water (about 25 seconds) until it runs clear. And you can mix and match different types of beans for more variety.

Shhhhhh . . . What About Gas?

Eliminate the gas factor by repeatedly soaking the dry beans and discarding the runoff. Do this repeatedly. Cook in fresh water. *Tip:* Soaking beans for 12 hours, then pouring off the water and cooking with fresh water should significantly reduce the amount of gas-producing compounds. And, if you're starting to add fiber to your diet, begin with a small dose so your bowel gets used to it.

With the use of fiber from grains, fruits, vegetables, legumes you are able to boost detoxification and strengthen your immune system against invaders!

— *HIGHLIGHTS* —

1. *Meet fiber, a powerful cell cleanser and waste remover.*

2. *Nicholas U. controlled cholesterol level and detoxified his bloodstream in nine days with the help of fiber. Remember to include California figs for a tasty source of fiber.*

3. *Only ten cents a day buys you enough bran for inner cleansing. It corrected Oliver E. K.'s problem of irregularity and digestive distress in a few days.*

4. *The "Morning Bran Tonic" revitalized Joan McC. within three days and helped her overcome slowness. She became a youthfully efficient worker.*

5. *Wheat germ is a tasty nugget of packaged health that brims with fiber. Use it daily for around-the-clock cellular detoxification.*

6. *Discover the little-known source of fiber and other nutrients—legumes! They will detoxify speedily, lower cholesterol, and protect against diabetes, says a physician.*

Chapter 17

OVERCOME HEMORRHOIDS, ULCERS, VARICOSE VEINS WITH NUTRITIONAL CLEANSING

Congestion, irritation, wastes: when locked in stagnant pools, they erupt in distressful disorders that require cleansing and detoxification. With better self-care, you can wash out congestion and restore free circulation to your internal organs. You can overcome some of the conditions or reactions traced to toxic overload.

HOW TO DETOXIFY YOUR HEMORRHOIDS

While hemorrhoids may be the source of snickers and giggles, they are not funny to the more than 25 million people who have this condition—at least one adult in every three households. They are no laughing matter. They are the result of toxemia.

What Are Hemorrhoids?

A network of hemorrhoidal veins is located in the lower area of the rectum at the junction with the anal canal. These veins are specialized vascular cushions and are directly affected by bowel movements. Constipation, diarrhea, and abrasive wastes can irritate the cushions, building up toxins and causing them to swell and bulge from beneath the thin layer of tissue that covers them. Blood fills the distended, ballooning cushions, forming tender, painful hemorrhoids.

Are There Different Types of Hemorrhoids?

There are two basic types: internal and external. Most individuals with hemorrhoids have both types in varying degrees.

1. *Internal hemorrhoids* occur in the upper portion of the anal canal and may cause pain, burning, itching, or an aching sensation. Bright red

blood on the stool or toilet tissue after a movement may mean internal hemorrhoids are present. They can be pushed down the anal canal during movements and protrude through the anus. These protruding or "prolapsed" hemorrhoids usually return spontaneously to their original position. If they remain prolapsed, they can become extremely painful and help is needed.

2. *External hemorrhoids* occur under the surface of the skin at the anal opening. They tend to disappear after a few days but frequently recur. They result from disruption of the spongy tissue of a superficial hemorrhoidal vein. This produces pain and swelling, burning and itching of the overlying skin. If severe pain or infection develops, help is needed.

What Are Symptoms of Hemorrhoids?

Pain, itching, burning, and swelling are the most common symptoms. Other symptoms include an aching sensation and a low backache or full feeling, particularly with internal hemorrhoids and blood on the stool. A health practitioner should be consulted if continuous or severe pain or bleeding occurs: this may be associated with a more serious condition.

What Causes Hemorrhoids?

Stress and pressure on the network of relatively delicate hemorrhoidal veins is a major cause. Straining during bowel movements and constipation can damage the hemorrhoidal cushions and cause the tissues to swell. Other causes include lifting heavy objects, violent coughing or sneezing, and sitting or standing for prolonged periods.

Is Constipation a Cause?

Constipation is a symptom of internal toxic overload. There is straining during bowel movements. As a result, poor blood flow or "venous back pressure" occurs, with blood-filled toxic wastes being "trapped" inside the hemorrhoidal veins. The stagnation causes blood clots to form in the swollen, inflamed hemorrhoidal tissue, leading to pain, itching, and bleeding. The person dreads the prospect of a bowel movement. This fear can lead to constipation, thus beginning the cycle again.

Who Gets Hemorrhoids?

Those who live in our modern society are especially prone to hemorrhoids. It is the result of a refined diet and sedentary lifestyle. This combination of diet and our tendency to ride, sit, and stand for long periods of time can lead to accumulation of toxins and bouts of hemorrhoidal symptoms.

Can Hemorrhoids Be Overcome?

There are detoxification steps to be taken to lessen the chance of hemorrhoids occurring or to keep them from becoming more serious. These include:

1. *Nutritional Cleansing.* Sweep away toxic overload with an increase in dietary fiber—the plant food not broken down during digestion. Good sources include minimally processed whole grain breads and cereals. Legumes (such as peas and beans) and millet (a grass), are excellent sources, as are root vegetables such as potatoes and carrots. *Super Cleansers:* California figs, bran, brown and wholemeal flours, brown and wholemeal breads, bran and wheat cereals, apples and pears with peels. Eat a variety of these fiber foods daily and start sweeping out wastes from your veins.

2. *Water or Liquids Detoxify Wastes.* Drink a minimum of six large glasses of liquid throughout the day. This is especially important when boosting fiber which tends to swell and absorb much moisture. Include caffeine-free beverages as well as fruit and vegetable juices as part of your liquid-detoxification program each day. Softer stools make it easier to detoxify your bowels and lessen pressure on the veins.

3. *Establish Regularity.* Obey the urge. Don't sit on the toilet too long. This is the only time the anus truly relaxes, allowing veins to fill with blood. The longer you sit, the longer pressure is put on the hemorrhoids. Reduce straining. Detoxify with high fiber foods to produce wastes that are softer and easier to pass. *Tip:* Establish a routine. Use the bathroom at the same time every day, particularly after a meal when the digestive process is naturally stimulated. It helps the bowel to adjust to a regular schedule.

4. *Keep Rectal Area Clean.* Washing, rinsing, drying should be done gently to protect this sensitive area.

5. *Exercise Regularly.* Exercise gives better tone to the supporting muscles of the ano-rectal area, as well as the abdomen as a whole. Additionally, by increasing the movement of food through the body, exercise helps protect against constipation. Brisk walking and other aerobic exercises help loosen toxic wastes and prepare them for elimination from congested tissues.

HOME CARE FOR HURTING HEMORRHOIDS

Soothing Sitz Bath. Sitting on a folded bath towel with a few inches of warm—not hot—water for 15 minutes, three or four times a day, or as your health practitioner may suggest, may help ease pain by relaxing muscles and soothing the hurtful area. The warm water soothes the pain and stimulates detoxification by increasing the flow of blood to the area, which in turn can help shrink the swollen veins.

Sit on a Doughnut. That is, a doughnut-shaped cushion to reduce pressure. They are useful if you must sit for long periods. Such cushions are available in pharmacies, medical supply stores, and many health stores.

Lose That Overweight. Excess poundage causes congestion and pressure on the lower extremities and more of a risk of problems with hemorrhoids. Shed those extra weighty pounds and you'll ease problems.

Soothe Hurt With Witch Hazel. If you have bleeding from external hemorrhoids, apply a dab of witch hazel to the area with a clean cotton ball. It causes blood vessels to contract. You might apply ice-cold witch hazel with the cotton ball, let it remain until no longer cold, then repeat. This herbal contains tannin which acts as an astringent.

CASE HISTORY—**Detoxifies Hemorrhoids, Enjoys Relief From Embarrassing Pain**

Edward LeC. felt "all shook up" after hours on the road as a deliveryman for a large wholesaler. He drove a tractor-trailer and bounced up and down on the road. When he developed hurtful tissues that made sitting painful, he worried about having hemorrhoids. He sought help from a urologist who suggested a program of detoxification to nip the problem in the bud. Edward LeC. started by planning more frequent rest stops. Then he would "fiber up" by eating more roughage from whole grain cereals, peas, beans, figs, and fruits (with peels) and by drinking lots of liquids. He also lost some excess weight. When he felt much discomfort, he would soothe the area with witch hazel which he applied during frequent rest stops. He tried not to sit or stand for extended periods. Whenever possible, he would keep physically active. Within three weeks, the hemorrhoids were "detoxified" and he could work in comfort . . . but he still maintained his inner cleansing program of high fiber foods and better self-care.

Hemorrhoids—they're no laughing matter . . . and no cause for embarrassment. With detoxification, you can heal the hurt and enjoy more comfort in your intimate zones.

HOW TO DETOXIFY YOUR ULCERS

An ulcer is a sore. There are two basic types of ulcers: A peptic ulcer is a sore in the stomach lining. A duodenal ulcer is a sore in the first part of the small intestine into which the stomach empties.

Symptoms include a gnawing pain between the breastbone and navel, ranging from mild to intense. The most common dangers arise from ulcers that bleed or perforate the stomach or duodenal wall. Bleeding occurs when the ulcer penetrates the muscular layer and ruptures blood vessels. Immediate medical care is required.

To help you correct toxemia and promote inner cleansing, a set of step-by-step suggestions is offered by Jon I. Isenberg, M.D., professor of medicine, University of California, San Diego School of Medicine:

"An important fact the patient can take home is that having ulcer disease does not alter survival, or mean being a life-long invalid who must eat nothing but bland, creamy foods. Regrettably, this notion persists despite efforts emphasizing it is unnecessary." Dr. Isenberg emphasizes, "Thinking in terms of what you can *do*, rather than what you *cannot* do, may enhance the ability to cope with flare-ups of acute ulcer. The best way to cope is to keep on doing, with few exceptions, all the things that contributed to a feeling of well-being before the diagnosis was made." Here is the doctor's inner cleansing program for ulcer detoxification:

1. Stop smoking. It contributes substantially to the incidence of cancer, respiratory and heart diseases, and is associated with peptic ulcer disease. In smokers, peptic ulcers occur more commonly, tend to heal more slowly, have more complications, and are more likely to require surgical treatment than nonsmokers. Said another way, a nonsmoker's peptic ulcer, properly treated, should heal in six to eight weeks. In a smoker, an ulcer of the same size and severity may take longer to heal. That leaves the smoker at a greater risk of complications, on the basis of healing time alone.

2. Avoid aspirin. It damages the stomach lining and can cause ulcers in the stomach. Eliminate all self-medication with products containing aspirin. More than a hundred over-the-counter products for everyday ills like upper respiratory infection and indigestion contain aspirin. Ulcer patients need to be told—over and over again—that aspirin is *bad* for ulcers. Enteric-coated aspirin causes less damage from direct irritation to the stomach, but after its absorption it may still have harmful systemic effects. To avoid aspirin in common medications, read the fine print on the package under "active ingredients" or ask the pharmacist.

3. Be careful about nonsteroidal anti-inflammatory drugs used to treat arthritis. They may damage the stomach lining, cause erosions and ulcers, and worsen ulcer disease. In this event, your physician can usually change medication schedules or reduce individual doses to overcome the problem.

4. A potentially harmful remedy is the regular use of baking soda—sodium bicarbonate—which is a potent neutralizer of acid. If used repetitively, it delivers an overload of sodium. The body then retains water, which may increase blood pressure or exacerbate heart disease. CAUTION: habitually ingesting sodium bicarbonate and drinking milk can cause the milk-alkali syndrome. This has a serious array of symptoms including raising blood calcium, causing calcium-containing kidney stones, and kidney failure.

5. Drinking alcohol in moderation has not been shown to cause ulcers or to prevent them from healing. However, chronic use of alcohol can cause gastritis, which mimics ulcer symptoms.

6. What about food? Let's challenge myths such as the need for a bland diet and avoidance of spicy foods, such as:

• Meat is not necessarily ulcerogenic, although it may cause fat buildup.

• Spicy foods do not cause or aggravate ulcers. Certain ethnic groups who consume great quantities of red-hot peppers are no more prone to peptic ulcer disease than any other group.

• Milk is not a medical treatment. While it does temporarily relieve the pain by neutralizing acid, it is a potent stimulant of acid production, thereby perpetuating the need for further neutralizing.

• Many ulcer patients claim that one food or another exacerbates their pain. To them I would say, avoid *anything* that causes you distress, as long as you remain on a balanced diet. Avoiding particular foods will not in itself enhance healing.

• Maintain a normal, three-meals-a-day schedule. Frequent small meals continuously stimulate the stomach to produce acid and pepsin. Having a snack at bedtime may even cause sleep-disrupting pain.

7. What about stress and ulcers? There is no convincing evidence that stress causes ulcers. The major problem is that it is difficult to quantify stress and the causes of stress vary from one person to another. Avoiding fear or anxiety-provoking stress whenever possible, is a good thing for ulcer people to do. But the same is surely true for everybody else as well. I know of absolutely no reason to tell ulcer patients to avoid excitement or exhilarating stress. Stress for one person may be

tranquility for others. Many people thrive on it; many others would give a lot—perhaps even risk an ulcer—to experience it.

8. As for antacids and other self-medications, discuss these with your physician. Over-the-counter remedies may intensify or diminish the effect of prescription drugs. Some antacids, for example, can impair the absorption of other drugs such as antibiotics.

Dr. Isenberg adds that with these guidelines, you will be able to cope with your condition. "Having a peptic ulcer today does not need to signal the end of a pleasant, satisfying, and worthwhile life."[28]

HOW TO DETOXIFY YOUR VARICOSE VEINS

Varicose veins are technically described as "saccular dilation of the veins which are often tortuous." The condition can be further defined as veins overburdened with toxic wastes, dilated beyond normal diameter and elongated beyond normal length. As a consequence of these anatomical aberrations, the vein has lost its normal function, which is to convey blood back to the heart.

Why? Because You're Human, That's Why They Happen!

Animals that walk on four legs don't get varicose veins, but people do. The upright human posture places great burdens on the vessels that must transport blood against the pull of gravity back to the heart, sometimes over a distance of almost five feet. They are an inevitable result of upright standing, poor posture, lack of exercise, overweight, restrictive clothing, excessive sitting, and refined foods. Toxic overload takes its toll in approximately one in five women and one in fifteen men by giving them stretched and swollen veins in their legs.

Checklist of Symptoms

Bluish, swollen, lumpy-looking veins and the crimson "spider veins" are only the most visible signs of this condition. Other symptoms include dull aching, heaviness, or swelling in the involved leg. Calf muscle cramps, occurring especially at night, are another recurring symptom. So is itching or a burning sensation over a prominent varicosity.

While not life-threatening, your entire body (especially your legs) will be much better off with a detoxification program following these six steps:

1. *Boost Fiber Intake.* More roughage makes regularity a comfortable occurrence. Otherwise, hard stools that result from a low-fiber or refined diet and the straining applied to eliminate them put excessive pressure on your leg veins. Include whole grains, legumes such as beans and peas, crisp vegetables, fruits with edible seeds (berries), and vegetables with edible stems or stalks (broccoli).

2. *Take a Walk.* Too much sitting could predispose a person to varicosities, says Howard Baron, M.D., vascular surgeon at New York University College of Medicine. "I call it 'the sitting disease.' Sitting virtually stills what is often called 'the venous or peripheral heart,' the muscular action in the legs that pumps blood back into your heart." Reason: If you're sitting, your leg muscles are not contracting, so your venous blood obeys the law of gravity. When blood pools in your legs, it builds up dangerous pressure in congenitally weak veins. You need to walk . . . walk . . . walk . . . more . . . more!

3. *Healthy Legs Still at Risk.* Ever experience the pins and needles feeling in your legs after sitting too long in one position? It's probably caused by a temporarily toxic or sluggish circulation that calls for prompt cleansing.

4. *Does a Chair Help?* Dr. Baron explains, "A chair puts unremitting pressure on the backs of the thighs, compressing the veins. The kinked veins at the knees and hips further build resistance to flow." Any stress on the vein walls is doubled when you sit in a chair; the pressure in your ankles is 250 times greater in a chair than if you sat on the floor.

5. *Get a Move On!* "Exercise, walk, run, jump, anything," urges Dr. Baron. "Anything that keeps your legs moving and your circulation going." He recommends perpetual motion, even if you're seated. "At your desk or crammed into an airline seat, you can still flex your calf muscles to get your venous heart pumping. Press your feet against the floor or, on an airplane, on the seat bar. Start wiggling your toes against the floor. Get up every hour or so and walk. If you're on an airplane, walk up and down the aisles. It's a good argument for flying coach. It's a longer walk," says the vascular surgeon.

6. *Loosen Tight Garments.* Constriction or compression of the legs by tight knee-high boots, garters, girdles, and panty hose or by crossing the legs while sitting can aggravate varicose veins, notes the doctor. He also suggests wriggling your toes frequently and periodically rising up on your toes should you be stuck in one spot for long. Don't wear binding garments around your groin or below. And also, not only

should you keep your legs uncrossed but put your feet up whenever possible.[29]

INNER CLEANSING FOR YOUR LEG VEINS

Here are some suggestions considered helpful in promoting better circulation and boosting inner cleansing of your leg veins:

1. When on a long plane or train trip, get up and walk around every 30 minutes. Or on a long trip by car, stop once in a while and get out to stretch your legs.

2. When you are reading (this book, for example) or watching television, elevate your feet. Rest your legs on a chair or stool. It's important to get your legs higher than your heart so they can properly detoxify.

3. Exercise is a great way to detoxify. Movements of leg muscles help push the blood upward. Swimming or walking in deep water is another helpful inner cleanser; the pressure of the water against your legs helps move blood up your veins.

4. Sleeping with your feet raised slightly above the level of your heart helps the blood flow away from your ankles. (This is not advisable for some people; check with your health practitioner.) If you have serious congestion, raise your bed by placing 6-inch-high blocks under the bedposts at the foot. This gives better support than simply raising the mattress.

5. For those confined to bed, movement of feet or legs should be encouraged to help circulation.

6. Round garters should never be worn. They cut off the venous circulation, thus raising pressure in the veins and increasing the risk of varicosities.

7. Elastic girdles should not be worn continuously—especially when you will be seated for a long time, such as at a desk, or during a plane, train, or auto trip. They bunch up and hamper the return of blood. This increases the pressure of the blood in the veins and worsens the toxemia of varicose veins.

8. Pregnant patients are advised to wear elastic stockings and to lie down occasionally during the day. Getting up soon after giving birth is also important.

9. It's important to get your legs higher than your heart, so the veins can properly detoxify. An easy way to do this is to lie on the floor and put

your feet up on a chair or couch. About 20 minutes of this detoxification program, repeated twice a day, is most helpful.

10. Discuss support hose with your health practitioner. They may need to be prescribed. They are helpful in resisting the blood's tendency to pool in the small blood vessels closest to the skin. Instead, the blood is cleansed and pushed into the larger, deeper veins, where it is more easily pumped back up to the heart.

Troubled with varicose veins? Don't just sit there—detoxify with these inner cleansing programs and enjoy overall better health.

───────────────── *HIGHLIGHTS* ─────────────────

1. *Detoxify the causes of hemorrhoids with a set of programs that wash out congestion.*
2. *Edward LeC. was able to overcome hurtful hemorrhoids with a nutritional program and the use of soothing witch hazel applications.*
3. *A leading physician offers an eight-step plan to detoxify your ulcers and heal much of the hurt.*
4. *Cleanse debris from your veins and overcome varicosities; those ugly bulges can be smoothed out through inner cleansing. A vascular surgeon offers a detoxifying program in six steps.*
5. *Inner cleanse your legs with better living practices as outlined.*

Chapter 18

HOW TO DETOXIFY YOUR DIGESTIVE SYSTEM AND BE FREE OF CONSTIPATION, DIARRHEA, STOMACHACHE

The digestive tract is a complex system of organs responsible for converting the food you eat into the nutrients you need to sustain your body and mind. You would expect a system as well used as the digestive tract to be the source of many toxic problems—and it is. Toxemia of the digestive tract is responsible for causing the hospitalization of more people than any other group of disorders. With the newer knowledge of inner cleansing, much can be done about detoxifying your system to protect against a broad spectrum of digestive problems.

What Goes Wrong?

Changes that predispose to toxemia are usually minor. They include slower action of the muscles of the digestive system and reduced acid production. Changes in lifestyle interfere with the cleansing and working power of the digestive system. Refined foods, less exercise, poor eating habits, inadequate nutrients all deposit wastes on the organs involved in the process of digestion. For example, low intake of fiber (the part of the plant that is not digested) allows toxins to build up and cling to the vital organs, bringing on many reactions such as constipation, indigestion, and stomachache, to name a few. With inner cleansing, you can detoxify blockages and enjoy regularity and better health.

HOW TO DETOXIFY CONSTIPATION

This condition is defined as the infrequent and difficult passage of waste. There is no accepted rule for the correct number of daily or weekly bowel movements. "Regularity" may be twice-daily for some or two movements a week for others. Chronically postponing your answer to nature's call can cause a loss of normal bowel reflexes. Medications can also cause toxic overload. Antihistamines and decongestants make the stool drier, causing more difficult movements. Many drugs slow down movement in the intestinal tract.

Laxatives? Beware!

Laxatives can become addictive. You may become dependent upon them. You increase dosages until, finally, the intestine becomes so insensitive, it fails to work properly. There is a thinning of the muscular wall of the colon. Lacking muscle tone, the colon can no longer contract as it should, and you endure painful spasms.

The Diet Connection

Marvin Schuster, M.D., chief of the division of digestive diseases, Baltimore (Maryland) City Hospitals, offers this set of guidelines for inner cleansing:

"Instead of relying upon laxatives and enemas, eat a well-balanced diet that includes unprocessed bran, whole wheat bread, prunes and prune juices, as well as California figs and fig juices. Bowel habits are also important; set aside sufficient time after breakfast or dinner, or after morning beverage, to allow for undisturbed visits to the toilet. And never ignore the urge!

"To stimulate intestinal activity, drink plenty of fluids and exercise regularly. Special exercises may be necessary to tone up abdominal muscles after pregnancy, or whenever abdominal muscles are lax. And remember, whenever there is a significant or prolonged change in your bowel habits, check with your doctor."[30]

EIGHT STEPS TO REGULARITY AND INNER CLEANSING

The U.S. Public Health Service explains that if no intestinal disease or abnormality exists and your health practitioner approves, try this eight-step detoxification program for correction of constipation:

1. Eat more fresh fruits and vegetables, either cooked or raw, and more whole grain cereals and breads. Dried fruits such as apricots, prunes, and California figs are especially high in fiber. Try to cut back on highly processed foods (such as refined sweets) and foods high in fat.

2. Drink plenty of liquids (1 to 2 quarts daily) unless you have heart, circulatory, or kidney problems. Be aware that some people become constipated from drinking large quantities of milk.

3. Some doctors recommend adding *small* amounts of unprocessed bran ("miller's bran") to baked goods, cereals, and fruits as a way of increasing the fiber content of your diet. If you eat a well-balanced diet with a variety of foods high in natural fiber, it usually is not necessary to add bran. But if you *do* use unprocessed bran, remember you may have bloating and gas for a few weeks after adding bran to your diet. All changes should be made slowly to allow your digestive system to adapt. And be sure to drink more liquids to protect against the gassy feeling of bran.

4. Stay active. Even taking a brisk walk after dinner can help tone your muscles.

5. Try to develop regular bowel habits. If you have had problems with constipation, attempt to have a bowel movement shortly after breakfast or dinner.

6. Avoid taking laxatives if at all possible. Although they will usually relieve the constipation, you become addicted to them and the natural muscle actions will be impaired.

7. Limit your intake of antacids, as some can cause constipation as well as other health problems.

8. Above all, do not expect to have a bowel movement every day or even every other day. "Regularity" differs from person to person. If your bowel movements are usually painless and occur regularly (whether the pattern is three times a day or two times each week), you are probably not constipated.[31]

CASE HISTORY—**Corrects Laxative Addiction**
With Simple Detoxification

A hectic schedule involving a family and part-time job, not to mention social obligations kept Lila V. J. always on the move . . . but not her bowels! She neglected "roughage" or fiber foods and habitually ate "fast foods" that built up her toxic waste overload. Her vital organs became clogged. She felt she had "no time" for a carefully planned food program and so reached for harsh laxatives. They so weakened her colon walls, she had to double the dose of laxatives and developed colitis, not to mention digestive backup. Lila V. J. realized she was headed for toxemia and its accompanying difficulties. She sought help from an internist who outlined an inner cleansing program to wash out the wastes that were blocking her vital functions. The eight-step program was followed, along with more healthful foods—more natural foods for better bulk and roughage. She was told to stop taking any laxatives. "Let your colon work by its own force," advised the doctor. Lila V. J. followed the eight-step program . . . and in eleven days, she was "regular" again. She no longer complained of irregularity! She had detoxified her digestive system . . . naturally.

HERBS THAT SCRUB AWAY WASTES

Certain herbs are able to detoxify your digestive system and promote regularity. These are available at most health stores or herbal pharmacists. They each have a beneficial scrubbing action that cleanses your internal organs to relieve constipation and related toxemia.

> *Flaxseed.* Make an infusion of crushed flaxseed and drink one cup of the "potion" in the morning and another in the evening.
>
> *Licorice Root.* Use the herb, *not* the commercial licorice which is artificial and sugary. Chew the root for inner cleansing. Or make a decoction of 1 teaspoon root in 1 cup of boiled water; drink one cup in the morning, another at noon, and a third at night.
>
> *Rose Hips Tea.* Make a decoction or infusion with halved rose hips; strain through filter paper to remove the seeds which could be irritating. Drink whenever necessary.

WATER: IMPORTANT CLEANSER

It is vital for you to drink enough water. Otherwise, your body will absorb more of the water from your colon to meet its needs, making the wastes difficult to uproot. As a general rule, drink six to eight glasses of water or its equivalent daily, and more if you are physically very active and sweat a lot. CAUTION: Alcohol and caffeinated beverages tend to be dehydrating, so for the sake of your digestive system, avoid them.

When Nature doesn't call regularly, take steps to detoxify and cleanse away blockages for correction of the problem.

HOW TO DETOXIFY DIARRHEA

Diarrhea is a condition in which body wastes are discharged from the bowel more often than usual and in a more or less liquid state. If it persists for weeks, it is an indication of severe illness. There may be other warning symptoms such as fever, abdominal cramps, weight loss, nausea and vomiting.

Diarrhea often represents the body's effort to detoxify itself or some noxious wastes. Normally, the large intestine (colon, lower bowel) absorbs water from solid wastes passed along by the small intestine. Diarrhea results when excessive toxins accumulate and interfere with that absorption; the bowel secretes rather than absorbs liquids.

Don't Neglect Diarrhea

Diarrhea may not "go away" by itself. The hazard is loss of water and body salts needed for normal cell function. Dehydration and salt imbalance can result in heart-rhythm disorders, blood pressure irregularity, kidney failure. Diarrheal illness can be fatal. For chronic diarrhea, see your health practitioner without delay.

Simple Steps to Ease Diarrhea

There are a number of programs to ease the distress and help remedy the problem.

- If you have repeated, unexplained bouts of diarrhea, stop using milk products for one or two weeks. You may have an insufficient amount of the enzyme *lactase* which digests milk sugar. To overcome this disorder, pretreat milk with the enzyme (available in health stores and pharmacies) or take milk-digestant tablets (also in health stores and pharmacies) before you consume milk products.
- Certain sugar substitutes such as mannitol or sorbitol found in dietetic products and sugarless gums can cause diarrhea if consumed to excess. If this is your situation, you would do well to avoid them.
- You may have a bacterial cause such as a toxin-producing strain of salmonella or food poisoning. Symptoms may persist for 24 hours or up to a week. (You should consult a physician at once). Your body is trying to detoxify.
- Stressful or tension-filled? An emotionally induced increase in the muscular contractions of your bowel can bring on diarrhea. You need to anticipate stress and cope with it in advance to minimize symptoms.

HOME REMEDIES FOR DETOXIFICATION OF DIARRHEA

Ease the situation with some of these detoxification remedies.

Herbal Tea. The soothing warmth is said to be comforting; herbs also contain an astringent, believed to protect the internal membranes from irritating toxemia. Herbal tea helps uproot and wash out these wastes.

Continue With Liquids. Increase fluid intake to replace that which is lost and ward off dehydration.

Carrot Juice Replaces Lost Nutrients. Carrot juice helps replace electrolytes and minerals lost during diarrhea. One or two glasses daily will be helpful.

Avoid Bubble Trouble. Any carbonated beverages should be avoided. They contain bubbly gas which adds abusive explosiveness to an already sensitive situation.

Is It Celiac Sprue? Diarrhea is a symptom of celiac sprue in which gluten (a protein found in some grains) hurts the lining of the small intestine and causes malabsorption of foods. If you have this disorder, avoid gluten-containing wheat, rye, barley, and malt. Switch to corn, brown rice, and oats.

Diarrhea is often referred to as "too much of a good thing." While inner cleansing is important, be alert to excessive loss and take steps to control your detoxification so that you have "enough of a good thing '

HOW TO DETOXIFY STOMACHACHE

"I have a terrible stomach ache. What can I do?" And that's just one expression of it. Except for the common cold, nothing is so troublesome for so many people in so many ways as an upset stomach. Call it indigestion, dyspepsia, gas, or heartburn, it is not at all pleasant. While not life-threatening, an upset stomach has annoying symptoms such as a sense of fullness or distention, gas, upper abdominal pain, general discomfort.

Why Does It Happen?

The delicate motions of the stomach and small intestine are regulated by your brain and by a network of nerves embedded in the muscle wall of the digestive tract. The coordination between these nerve endings that secrete a variety of chemical substances (called neurotransmitters), hormones, and the muscle fibers in the wall of the digestive tract all regulate the movement of the tract. This process promotes the digestion, absorption, and elimination of the food you eat. Any disruption in the normal functioning of the nervous system or the muscular activity of the digestive tract can cause stomach upset. It tends to be more common in women.

What are some of the disruptions that cause distress? They also deposit toxic wastes that get your signals crossed and lead to an ache. These include:

- *Fatty Foods.* They clog your metabolic channels and slow down your stomach's normal activities. Excessive intake of fat can inhibit stomach digestion and deposit wastes on your vital organs that clog free transportation of nutrients and oxygen.

- *Emotional upset.* Anger, resentment, and anxiety accelerate stomach acid secretions causing "acid stomach." Some acid may be transported via a gas bubble into your esophagus, bringing on distress.

- *Fast eating.* Gobbling your food interferes with natural assimilation, and you run the risk of toxic overload and stomach distress.

- *Air swallowing.* When extreme, the problem of aerophagia can bring on such reactions as abdominal distention, smothering sensations, palpitations.

- *Spicy foods.* For some, too much seasoning can irritate the stomach lining and cause distress. Check your reactions, does too much seasoning cause distress? If so, use herbal flavorings in moderation. More is not necessarily better.

- *Pre-meal stress.* Strain from tension and nervousness prompt the stomach to secrete excessive amounts of acid. If no food is present to break down, the acid irritates the stomach lining. If you are under constant strain, plan to give yourself 30 to 60 minutes of relaxation before you eat.

ANTACIDS: MORE HARM THAN GOOD

The California Medical Association tells us, "For many people, the symptoms of indigestion may be prevented simply by improved eating practices and reduction of emotional tension.

"Over-the-counter antacids are sometimes effective in the treatment of indigestion, but can be over-used and may produce undesirable side effects. Over-the-counter antacids contain at least one of several acid neutralizing chemicals.

"While providing some relief of gas and pain, some antacids also contain high amounts of sodium, calcium, aluminum, manganese, and even sugar. Used over a long period of time, some of these substances can be harmful and upset the body's acid balance.

"Some antacids can cause constipation or acid rebound, which is an increase in the production of stomach acid after the antacid effect has worn off. Sodium bicarbonate can cause several problems and should rarely be taken as an antacid.

"Furthermore, antacids may interfere with the action of some drugs such as tetracycline antibiotics, iron, arthritis medicines and some heart medicines, some medications for psychiatric disorders and many others. You are advised to consult with your physician before taking any type of antacid." [32]

DETOXIFICATION HINTS, TIPS, SUGGESTIONS

- Food combinations are important. Milk should not be consumed with meals. Starches and proteins are not a good combination. Sugars should not be consumed with starches or proteins.
- Sip one tablespoon of pure apple cider vinegar in a glass of water with meals to help detoxify wastes and improve digestion.
- First thing in the morning, drink the juice of a small lemon in a cup of freshly boiled water. It helps cleanse the bloodstream of sediment.
- Broth made out of either brown rice or barley will give your clogged organs a scrubbing and ease disorders such as heartburn, bloating, and gas. To prepare, use five parts water to one part grain. Boil for 10 minutes. Let simmer another 45 minutes. Strain, cool and sip at intervals throughout the day.
- Boost detoxification with dandelion tea. Collect the small leaves of the dandelion plant. (The larger leaves are too bitter.) Wash and place them in boiling water in a covered stainless steel pot. Steep until leaves are tender. Add a few mint leaves to flavor and honey to taste. Sip a small cup of the hot beverage after meals.
- Peppermint or spearmint tea is soothing and also cleansing, especially if you are troubled with a digestive disorder.

Detoxify your digestive system and enjoy a healthier lifestyle. After all, good health begins with clean digestion!

——————————— *HIGHLIGHTS* ———————————

1. *Detoxify constipation with natural remedies.*
2. *Inner cleansing of your entire digestive system is possible with an official eight-step detoxification program. Easy, effective, energizing.*
3. *Lila V. J. overcame hurtful laxative addiction on a simple detoxification program easily followed at home.*

4. *Herbs are helpful in scrubbing away wastes that clog your digestive organs.*

5. *Simple steps detoxify diarrhea, a condition not to be ignored.*

6. *Detoxify stomachache with the simple changes described.*

7. *Regenerate your digestive system with the easily followed detoxification hints and tips.*

Chapter 19

THE RAW JUICE WAY TO SUPER CLEANSING AND HEALTHY YOUTH AT ANY AGE

Fresh fruit and vegetable juices are powerhouses of nutrients that revitalize and regenerate your entire body and mind. These refreshing juices send forth cleansing catalysts that penetrate the innermost recesses of your body and dislodge accumulated grit and pollutants from your cells and organs. At the same time, the juices use their rich endowment of nutrients to repair your vital tissues and organs to give you the look and feel of youth, no matter what your age.

CAUSE OF AGING: CELLULAR TOXEMIA

To understand the importance of cleansing with raw juices, you need to know the real cause of aging and how to reverse this threat. Aging occurs when the biological process of cell regeneration becomes sluggish. What causes this slowdown? Toxemia: the accumulation of grime and sediment in your tissues. These pollutants prevent cellular nourishment. Denied essential elements, your cells starve; they wither and die. This is the root cause of aging.

Cells Need Cleansing and Nourishment

You are a magnificent package of cells. Each one is an independent unit with its individual metabolism. It needs to be kept clean and nourished. It must have a constant supply of life-giving oxygen. *Problem:* If there is any accumulation of rust-like plaque that clings to the membranes and cellular interior, there is a clogging of the flow of oxygen and nourishment. Cellular disintegration occurs. If too many of your cells die in the polluted overload, the aging process takes hold. You can see it in aging skin. You can feel it in tiredness and a weakened immune system. To nip this in the bud, you need to use juices to invigorate your cells with cleansing and nourishment and detoxification.

RAW JUICES ARE SWIFT IN CELLULAR REGENERATION

You need swift cellular detoxification. Your cells are in a constant dying-replacement process. If more cells break down and die than are rebuilt, the aging process strikes all the quicker. Aged and decaying cells decompose rapidly. To prevent their accumulation and clogging, you need to eliminate them as quickly as possible. *Remedy:* Fresh juices rebuild cells and wash out the decayed and dead leftovers so they do not accumulate and cause toxemia.

Cleanses, Rebuilds, Revitalizes

Within moments after you consume a glass of your favorite raw juice, the nutrients and enzymes go to work to create internal rejuvenation. The juice nutrients speed up the biological process of detoxifying the dead and decaying cells and washing them away. The juice nutrients then accelerate the building of new cells. When the toxic waste products that have been blocking cellular oxygenation and nourishment are washed out, then the juices stimulate metabolic and cell-rebuilding functions.

Juices Detoxify Faster Than Whole Foods

The extracted liquid portion of fruits or vegetables is a highly concentrated source of super cleansing without comparison. The juice is rapidly assimilated by your digestive system, requiring almost no digestive action. For this reason, you feel an instant "lift" when drinking a glass of orange juice, much swifter than if you eat the whole fruit.

Whole fruits and vegetables that are thoroughly chewed are extremely valuable sources of nutrients and detoxifying elements. Enjoy them daily for overall regeneration. But for swift action on cellular scrubbing, raw juices are the key. Together, the combination helps you enjoy a prolonged "prime of life" at any age

SEVEN CLEANSING-REJUVENATION POWERS OF FRESH JUICES

Fresh juices offer these immediate detoxification rewards via cleansing and rejuvenation.

1. *Nutritional Regeneration.* Free of the pulp, the rich juices contain high concentrations of vitamins, minerals, trace elements, and enzymes that work speedily to promote nutritional regeneration and detoxification of your body.

2. *Quick Assimilation.* In liquid form, these valuable cleansing elements are quickly assimilated into your bloodstream. As juices, they do *not* require digestive effort, hence their "instant" absorption and detoxification functions. These juices do not interfere with other digestive activities, and pose no "load" on your system.

3. *Bypass Hydrochloric Acid.* Fresh juices do not require hydrochloric acid, which often causes cellular disintegration, in excess. Spare your digestive system the outpouring of this harsh and volatile acid; juices are metabolized without distress or discomfort.

4. *Total Package of Detoxification.* The concentrated nutritive elements stabilize your basic biological processes so that detoxification is more effectively performed. Juice nutrients are so perfectly balanced by nature that they speed up the cleansing-regeneration process almost at the very start.

5. *Balances Acid-Alkaline Levels.* Vegetable juices are dynamic sources of alkaline reserve. This helps establish the important acid-alkaline balance in your bloodstream. Distress is eased. Corrosive wastes are washed away from your vital organs.

6. *Improves Mineral Nourishment.* Abundant supplies of minerals in the juices restore the biochemical and amino acid balance in your bloodstream, cells, tissues, organs. *Special Benefit:* A mineral deficiency precedes oxygen loss which could "choke" and "starve" your cells and allow waste buildup. With juices, minerals provide needed oxygen and nourishment and accelerate the detoxification process.

7. *Speeds Up Inner Cleansing.* Fresh raw juices are chock full of detoxifying enzymes which alert the *micro-electric tension factor* in your body. This speeds up inner cleansing. At the same time, this factor creates a "magnet" action whereby nutrients are absorbed from your bloodstream to nourish your internal organs. This same "magnet" action detoxifies by eliminating metabolic refuse.

The best indication of the cleansing-healing power of juices is felt when you finish one or two glasses of a freshly prepared beverage. You feel refreshed, alert, and good all over. This is the "instant" detoxification power of fresh juices.

Selecting Your Fruits, Vegetables

Produce should be fresh, seasonal, and free of decay. If you notice any signs of deterioration, just cut away that portion and discard.

Wash all fruits and vegetables before you juice them. Use free-flowing cold water from your kitchen faucet. If you prefer, use a scrub brush for your vegetable to make certain dirt and debris have been removed.

If possible, juice your fruits or vegetables the same day you bring them home from the market. Otherwise, store in the crisper of your refrigerator. Do *not* cut until ready to juice, since this causes loss of important cleansing nutrients.

Easy Way to Prepare Juice

You may use a manual juicer or an electric appliance. These are available at health stores and houseware outlets. Just cut up the fruit or vegetable and insert in your juicer. Plan to use the squeezed juice promptly. You may store it overnight in a closed container in your refrigerator, although a small amount of the nutrients will evaporate. Use squeezed juice within two days, though, to derive maximum detoxification benefits.

Do Not Combine Fruit With Vegetable Juice

Fruit enzymes and nutrients are of a different density than those found in vegetables. If combined, there is a diluting of these elements and the cleansing-regenerative abilities are weakened. Combining them is a "no-no."

Feel free to combine any seasonal fresh fruits, if desired, for a tasty juice that works without delay. Also, it is fine to combine different seasonal vegetables to make a powerful cleansing beverage.

SIMPLE JUICE-DETOXIFICATION PROGRAM

Plan to consume about three or four glasses of juice daily on this easy program. *Before breakfast:* a glass of fresh fruit juice. *Noontime:* a glass of fresh fruit juice. *Dinnertime:* a glass of fresh vegetable juice after your meal. *Nightcap:* a glass of fresh vegetable juice. This helps you sleep better, too, through comforting mineralization of your cells and tissues.

This simple juice-detoxification program nourishes your body, stimulates around-the-clock cleansing-regeneration to help you look and feel much younger and healthier.

CASE HISTORY—Erases 30 "Aging" Years for 30 Cents in Three Days

Crepe-like skin, hangdog look, poor memory, shaking hands and chronic fatigue made Ida DiN. fearful of having to look in the mirror. When someone erringly remarked she was her daughter's grandmother, she was spurred into action. She asked a health spa dietician for guidance on overcoming her premature aging. The dietician said countless people were able to roll back the clock on a detoxification raw juice fast. For three days she was to consume no food, but take only juices: the first day, all fruit juices, the second day, all vegetable juices, the third day, all fruit juices. Afterwards she was to gradually return to a healthful diet. Ida DiN. dragged herself to a nearby wholesaler and bought a supply of fresh produce. She began the program. Immediately, her skin firmed up, she sparkled with vitality, had improved memory, firm hands, and welcome energy. In only three days, she looked as if she had shed 30 years, and all for only 30 cents per day, the cost of the juices. Afterwards, she would frequently have a raw juice fast to detoxify. She had made herself brand new—inside and outside!

TASTY JUICES FOR HEALING OF COMMON AILMENTS

Everyday fruits and juices offer cleansing elements that stimulate quick healing of many common ailments. The juices are tasty. The results are amazingly effective.

Carrot Juice for Digestive System Detoxification

The rich concentration of beta-carotene, minerals, and fiber in carrot juice combine to swiftly speed up digestive-intestinal detoxification. These combined nutrients do more than liquefy and dilute wastes, they hasten their removal. These nutrients further boost bile acid removal and cleansing of the colon. Your digestive-eliminative system becomes detoxified and super-charged with vitality after you enjoy one or two glasses of carrot juice daily.

Intestine Cleanser

Cabbage juice contains factors that wash away the plaque clinging to your intestines. These same scrubbing factors dilute the hydrochloric acid and protect against ulcer formation and burning. Cabbage juice also detoxifies wounds in the stomach lining, helping to heal ulcerous infections.

Cool Internal Inflammation

Tangy cranberry juice detoxifies your bloodstream, helps acidify your urine to protect against *dysuria* (painful elimination) and disorders of the bladder and prostate gland. Painful voiding is eased when cranberry juice washes away irritating wastes and brings about a soothing and natural release.

CASE HISTORY—**Juice Cools Kidney Inflammation**

In a reported situation, a 66-year old woman, Mabel O'H. was troubled with kidney inflammation for several years. Diagnosed as chronic pyelonephritis, she submitted to drugs, antibiotics, and painful dilations—but with little improvement. She was put on a cranberry juice program, told to drink two six-ounce glasses daily. After eight weeks, her urine gradually began to clear. At the end of nine months, there was only occasional toxic debris. She continued on with the simple cranberry juice program because it helped her detoxify the cause of kidney inflammation when drugs did not.

Apple Juice as Virus-Cleanser

Fresh apple juice contains a virus-fighting substance that is able to detoxify dangerous germs. These substances combine with the virus during transit through the digestive system, help "knock it out," and then eliminate it. Several glasses of apple juice throughout the week help detoxify viral infestations and protect you against molecular deterioration caused by these substances.

Dissolve Mucus With Pineapple Juice

Freshly prepared pineapple juice contains a digestive enzyme called *bromelain*. This is a powerful mucus washer. It dissolves the mucus and prepares it for elimination. Mucus not only clogs your respiratory-bronchial tract, but also creates blockages in other parts of your body. It is toxic waste that clings together to weaken your immune system. With enzyme-powerful pineapple juice, you can discharge this waste.

CASE HISTORY—**Washes Away Gastric Wastes in Three Months**

At age 57, Rose A. Q. started to complain of after-dinner distress and bouts of colitis. Tests showed she had a thick accumulation of wastes in her stomach. (Diagnosed as a ball-like mass, it lodged in her digestive system.) Her physician had administered various chemical medications to dissolve the waste mass, but it caused so much burning, it had to be stopped. Then Rose A. Q. was told to take about 10 ounces of plain pineapple juice, three times a day, 30 minutes before each meal. In eight weeks, X rays showed the bezoar had shrunk to half its original size. A few weeks later, the threatening waste mass was gone! The mucus glue had been dissolved through the detoxifying power of the bromelain in the pineapple juice. She was healed. All this happened in less than three months.

Vegetable Juices Cleanse Toxic Bacteria

Eight vegetable juices contain a powerful detoxifying enzyme called *lysozyme*. When you drink juices made from these vegetables (singly or in any desired combination) you release the lysozyme waste cleanser, which seizes toxic bacteria and foreign particles and prepares them for expulsion. Once detoxified, you are rewarded with a cleaner and healthier body, free of harmful toxic bacteria. These eight vegetable juices are made from: cauliflower, cabbage, red radish, white radish, turnip, parsnip, broccoli, rutabaga. *Suggestion:* Blenderize these vegetables into a puree for a powerful detoxifying raw juice. The slight pulp in the puree provides sweeping fiber that doubles the cleansing action.

You *can* drink your way to a cleaner body and a healthier way of living. You can roll back the years as you wash out your wastes with raw juices, your rivers of super health.

HIGHLIGHTS

---

1. *Fresh raw juices cleanse your cells and organs to promote regeneration and rebuilding of your vital systems.*
2. *Note the seven cleansing-rejuvenating and detoxifying powers of fresh juices.*
3. *Ida DiN. washed away 30 years of aging for only 30 cents in juices in three days.*
4. *Mabel O'H. detoxified kidney inflammation on a cranberry juice program.*
5. *Rose A. Q. dissolved toxic lumps in her stomach and avoided surgery with the use of simple pineapple juice. All natural, all within three months.*

Chapter 20

A TREASURY OF CLEANSING PROGRAMS FOR EVERYDAY PROBLEMS

Everyday foods, simple exercises, inhalation, and tasty homemade tonics have the ability to dislodge the accumulated toxic wastes in your system and eliminate them. Once your vital organs and systems have been detoxified, you are able to enjoy speedy healing for many internal and external health disorders.

Here is a mini-treasury of everyday health problems that can be traced to toxic accumulation. The simple cleansers work almost at once. They help inner cleansing through detoxification so you enjoy effective healing and cleaner rejuvenation.

HIGH BLOOD PRESSURE

The use of garlic, one or two cloves daily as part of a salad or in cooking, helps control your pressure. Garlic has dilating effect on your blood vessels; it cleanses the blockages that prevent free blood flow and can cause arterial narrowing and a rise in blood pressure. Garlic is a great detoxifier to be used daily.

ACNE

Boost intake of foods and juices high in the cleansing vitamins A and D. These include fish, carrots, broccoli, sun-dried apricots, cantaloupe, and vitamin D-fortified skim milk. These vitamins cleanse the sebaceous glands of wastes that clog and plug skin pores, triggering blemishes.

ARTHRITIS

This disabling ailment is often traced to a nutritional imbalance and also to the accumulation of hurtful free radicals. Sediment blocks the metabolic process. Cleanse debris by taking antioxidant nutrients that clear away toxic free radicals; these include beta-carotene, C, E, zinc, and selenium.

ATHEROSCLEROSIS

Hardening of the arteries is caused by excessive fatty waste accumulation. Cleanse away debris with lecithin, a fat melting food (available in health stores) and more toxemia-washing fresh juices.

CASE HISTORY—Three-Day Artery Cleansing

Creeping atherosclerosis threatened to close in on her heart muscle so Bernice L. followed a detoxification program as outlined by her physician. She omitted all animal-source foods. She then took four tablespoons of waste-washing lecithin daily, in her vegetable juices, sprinkled over salads, added to her cereal, baked in meatless loaves, added to soups. Results? In three days, an examination showed she had "clean arteries." She had detoxified them with these simple inner cleansing methods.

RHEUMATIC INFLAMMATION

Similar to arthritis, the excessive throbbing heat is the result of chafing, irritating debris that clings to your skeletal and venous structures. To promote inner cleansing, include garlic in your daily food plan. *Simple:* Eat two or three carefully chewed garlic cloves daily; mask the odor with parsley, cloves, or cinnamon. Garlic is an excellent detoxifier; it boosts your metabolism, stimulates cleansing. It helps ease and erase the toxic cause of rheumatic fever, often in days.

SORES, WOUNDS

For swift detoxification, mix freshly grated garlic with olive oil as a poultice. Apply to sores or blemishes. Massage gently. The toxic-fighting ingredients in the garlic and the essential fatty acids of the olive oil cleanse away infectious bacteria and restore cellular integrity and swift healing. Repeat for several days.

BREATHING DIFFICULTIES

Whether an allergy, sensitivity, or congestion, you need to detoxify the accumulated wastes that are clinging to the delicate fibers of your respiratory organs. A simple detoxification remedy is to stand before an open window (be careful of drafts, though) and breathe in through your nostrils very deeply. Think of your lungs as balloons. Fill up to the brim! Hold for the count of 10. Then exhale slowly through your mouth. Repeat five times. This deep breathing helps sweep away toxic wastes that are choking your lungs and causing breathing difficulties.

MOUTH SORES

Fragile oral tissues split and break because the membranes have become clogged with wastes. You need to rebuild your mouth tissues. The use of bioflavonoids (in citrus fruits and their juices; eat the white membranous strings which are highly concentrated in these cleansing-rebuilding nutrients) will help heal this condition speedily.

FEVER BLISTERS

You need to detoxify the toxic waste clumps from these pus-filled blisters. *Remedy:* Dip a cotton swab into a bit of ether (from pharmacist) and apply to the blister. It "destroys" the toxic germs and helps remove them. Within moments, the blister or cold sore starts to heal.

CONSTIPATION

Weakened or inactive bowels become choked with stubborn toxic waste deposits. To cleanse, activate your sphincter muscles with all-natural prune or fig juice (or a combo). One or two glasses in the morning helps "knock out" the bacterial blockages and speed their removal. Try several California figs followed by a glass of any fruit juice for immediate detoxification in the morning.

CRAMPS

Whether in your arms, back, legs, or anywhere else, cramps can be debilitating. They indicate bacterial wastes are "locked in" your skeletal and musculature structures. A danger here is that they "devour" calcium which leads to cramps. To detoxify, drink several glasses of skim milk daily. The rich concentration of calcium helps strengthen these pockets and "chase" out wastes. In many situations, it works overnight!

CASE HISTORY—**Detoxifies Lifelong Cramps
With One Home Remedy**

Severe cramps, especially upon awakening, made Allen T. feel like an in-valid. It took him an hour to "untie the knots." But the pains always came back! A metabolic physician (specialist in whole body treatments) diagnosed toxemia—infectious wastes had lodged in muscular pockets and were caus-ing congestion. A simple remedy: boost intake of cleansing and restoring calcium through one or two glasses of skim milk, especially at night time. Allen T. tried it. Miraculously, the next morning, the pains were gone. Thanks to the detoxifying calcium, he overcame the cramps that had been plaguing him for a lifetime.

STRESS, TENSION

You know the symptoms: you cannot relax, you're high-strung, nervous, jumpy. The reason is that debris is grating and chafing at your nerves. Cleanse away this irritating toxemia and you feel soothed all over. Do this with a simple "rag doll" detoxification approach. Lie down in bed. Let your-self go. Concentrate on releasing all tightness from the tips of your fingers to the top of your head. Make yourself as limp as a dishrag. *Tip:* Your head should be able to roll easily from side to side. If you have any stiffness or resistance, you have not relaxed enough. Keep on making yourself limp. In so doing, tight pockets of wastes will be dislodged and washed out in a short time. Only 30 minutes daily of this "rag doll" detoxification and you free yourself from grating stress.

HEADACHES

Wash away irritating debris caused by caffeine and tannic acids by avoiding beverages and foods that contain them (coffee, commercial teas, colas, and chocolate). Switch to fresh fruit and vegetable juices. They contain detoxify-ing nutrients and cleansing enzymes that uproot and sweep away nerve-grating caffeine wastes.

STOMACH UPSET

One or two well-chewed garlic cloves helps create a magical soothing. Garlic is a prime source of a waste-cleanser known as *gasteoenteric allichalon* which washes away debris from the motor activation center of your stom-ach. Within moments, the detoxification restores comfort. It's a natural stomach tonic.

FOR WOMEN ONLY

Menstrual cramps and premenstrual syndrome need not be endured. Toxic wastes need to be removed. The hormonal influences of a monthly cycle are damaged if bacterial sludge becomes a piled up barrier. To detoxify these barricades, two remedies are effective. (1) In a glass of fresh fruit juice, add 1 tablespoon of brewer's yeast powder (from any health store). Stir vigorously or blenderize. Drink slowly. It is a powerhouse of enzymes, B-complex vitamins and vitamin C. They converge upon the wastes, then uproot and eliminate them. A soothing contentment is felt almost at once. (2) With the approach of the monthly period, wastes often gather together and displace valuable blood calcium. This mineral is a powerful pain reliever. Use calcium supplements or skim milk. Blood calcium levels are balanced quickly and wastes are washed out; contentment is restored.

RECTAL ITCHING

Blame this embarrassing problem upon venous congestion, especially wastes from white sugar and white flour products. Chemical residues accumulate in the veins and arteries of the groin and bring on a nagging itch. To correct, eliminate all foods containing sugar and bleached flour. A simple detoxification helps you become cleaner and itch-free almost at once.

ACID (SOUR) STOMACH

Often called heartburn. Blame it on excessive accumulation of acid-producing byproducts. Detoxify by avoiding alcohol, coffee, commercial tea, tobacco, and most animal-source foods. Try several baked or boiled potatoes daily—the potato stimulates an alkaline reaction in the body that helps neutralize stomach acidity and detoxify the irritating acidic wastes. Boost intake of potatoes (without salt or fatty dressing) and feel your stomach cleansing itself and becoming "sweet" again.

COLDS, WINTER AILMENTS

Clean those viral infections. For centuries, garlic has been used to ease problems such as sore throat, runny nose, fever, and cough. Just one or two garlic cloves daily helps detoxify your system and conquer your colds quickly. Also increase intake of detoxifying vitamin C through fresh fruits and juices.

HOW JUICES GIVE YOU QUICK CLEANSING AND BETTER HEALTH

Fresh fruit and vegetable juices are assimilated rapidly so their nutrients and enzymes can cleanse your cells and open channels for improved health. Here is a listing of various juices that will boost healing of many health disorders.

Apple Juice. Improves elimination; helps cleanse your bone structure; loosens blockages to correct digestive disorders.

Apricot Juice. A prime source of highly concentrated vitamins, minerals, and enzymes to purify the bloodstream and detoxify the circulatory system.

Beet Juice. Very potent, so combine with other vegetable juices such as celery, cucumber, lettuce, or cabbage. Its detoxifying action purifies your bloodstream, cleanses your nervous system.

Blackberry Juice. Combine with equal amounts of fresh water and drink in the morning to stimulate peristalsis, which then promotes regularity. A healthy cleanser.

Blueberry Juice. Its concentration of bioflavonoids helps stabilize your digestive system; soothes problems such as colitis, diarrhea, intestinal infections. *Tip:* When troubled with excessive amounts of uric acid, a waste product, drink a small amount of blueberry juice. It is a natural detoxifier of such waste.

Carrot Juice. Cleanses vital organs, neutralizes circulating blood impurities and also detoxifies skin blemishes. A prime source of beta-carotene (precursor of vitamin A) which improves your skin health.

Celery Juice. Drink it alone or mixed with other vegetable juices (with a squeeze of lemon or lime). It cleanses the liver and kidneys, detoxifies impurities of the bloodstream. Helps cleanse adrenal glands and scour components of the nervous system.

Cherry Juice. The unusually rich concentration of both bioflavonoids and enzymes make this a high-energy drink. Helps detoxify cells and tissues, protects against sludge-causing aging. Appears to protect against arthritis.

Cucumber Juice. A refreshing drink; its mildness should not be deceiving. Acts as a powerful solvent of uric acid, an undesirable waste. Drink it pure or combine with carrot and/or celery juices. Washes away debris in a matter of hours.

Currant Juice. Whether made from red or black currants, this juice is a powerful organ cleanser. Enzymes and nutrients detoxify wastes that might otherwise clog your liver and digestive organs.

Grape Juice. Rich in natural fruit sugars, it gives you youthful energy in minutes. Cleanses away impurities. Boosts excretion of urea, thereby detoxifying internal congestion. If you use bottled or canned grape juice, make certain it is free of added sugar.

Grapefruit Juice. Its powerful nutrients stimulate the flow of bile, improving the health of your liver. Cleanses tissues and cells so that wastes cannot destroy capillaries.

Lemon Juice. Very potent, so take only two or three tablespoons as part of a citrus juice combo. Its vitamin C and minerals detoxify blood impurities and protect against infectious allergies and respiratory distress.

Lettuce Juice. The rich concentration of cleansing nutrients helps detoxify wastes from organs to prevent spasms or grating irritation.

Orange Juice. The vitamins, minerals, and enzymes help cleanse blood plasma of impurities and strengthen vascular walls. Especially detoxifying are the bioflavonoids found in the pulp. Use it all.

Peach Juice. Prompts natural elimination to wash away stored-up wastes.

Pear Juice. Nutrients scrub intestinal organs and kidneys; the minerals regenerate your blood cells.

Pineapple Juice. A near-miracle juice rich in scrubbing enzymes that uproot the most stubborn of wastes. Powerful cleanser of vital organs.

Tomato Juice. It should be salt-free. Provides detoxifying nutrients that cleanse the bloodstream, revitalize the arteries and protect against cellular deterioration.

Easy Detoxification Plan

Take fresh juices daily for around-the-clock detoxification. The inner cleansing process works while you sleep. You will be rewarded with youthful immunity against illness and a lifestyle brimming with energy and vitality.

The headlines tell the story. You are subjected to a relentless assault on your health by a rain of toxic substances—from pesticides to prescription drugs, from caffeine to chemicals, from pollution in every breath you take.

You need to expel toxins from your body. You need to build immunity with the use of nutrition and fitness. You can fight back!

You can be healthier, look younger, and have a sparkling clean body—inside and outside. With these detoxification programs, you can enjoy a sludge-free, healthier life span.

Free yourself from joint-muscle-artery-circulation toxemia and enter a world of "eternal youth,"—beginning right now!

--------------------- *HIGHLIGHTS* ---------------------

1. *Clear up toxemia-related disorders with everyday foods and simple healers that promote internal-external cleansing in minutes.*

2. *Bernice L. overcame the risk of atherosclerosis with a simple three day artery-detoxification method.*

3. *Allen T. freed himself from his lifelong cramps battle with one home remedy that worked overnight.*

4. *Fresh juices are powerhouses in detoxifying your body and promoting youthful well-being. Refreshingly good, too.*

NOTES

1. Dr. Jack Soltanoff, West Hurley, New York, personal interview, July, 1991.

2. Benjamin Lau, M.D., *Garlic for Health*, Lotus Light Publications, Wilmot, Wisconsin, 1988, p. 25.

3. J. W. Anderson, M.D., *"Dietary Fiber, Lipids, Atherosclerosis*, Journal of Cardiology, Vol. 60, pp. 17G–22G, October 30, 1987.

4. Judith Stern, D.Sc., personal interview, April, 1991.

5. Kenneth Cooper, M.D., *Controlling Cholesterol*, Bantam Books, Inc., New York, New York, 1990, pp. 40–107.

6. Karen Burke, M.D., press bureau, May, 1991.

7. Douglas David Altchek, M.D., press interview, June, 1991.

8. Skin Cancer Foundation, press bureau, July, 1991.

9. Sun and Skin News, Vol. 7, No. 1, 1990, pp. 1, 4.

10. Edward Frohlich, M.D., press interview, June, 1991.

11. Stephen Brunton, M.D., press interview, July, 1991.

12. Ray Gifford, M.D., press interview, June, 1991.

13. Benjamin Lau, M.D., *Garlic for Health*, Lotus Light Publications, Wilmot, Wisconsin, 1988, pp. 17–19.

14. William Frishman, M.D., press interview, March, 1991.

15. Marvin Schuster, M.D., National Institutes of Health, press bureau, September, 1990.

16. Arthur Lubitz, M.D., press interview, June, 1991.

17. Lester Morrison, M.D., Dr. Morrison's Heart Saver Program, St. Martin's Press, New York, New York, 1982, pp. 83–84.

18. Dean Ornish, M.D., *Dr. Dean Ornish's Program To Reversing Heart Disease*, Random House, New York, New York, 1990, pp. 107–143.

19. Robert H. Garrison, Jr., M.A., R.Ph. and Elizabeth Somer, M.A., R.D., *Nutrition Desk Reference*, Keats Publishing Co., New Canaan, Connecticut, 1990, pp. 232–233.

20. Richard Kavner, O.D., *Total Vision*, A & W Publishers, New York, New York, 1978, pp. 135–157.

21. Joan Ullyot, M.D., personal interview, May, 1990.

22. Julian Whitaker, M.D., press bureau, February, 1990.

23. John W. Anderson, M.D., press bureau, May, 1989.

24. Rodolfo Paoletti, M.D., press interview, July, 1991.

25. Claude Lenfant, M.D., press interview, July, 1991.

26. Sheldon Hendler, M.D., *Complete Guide to Anti-Aging Nutrients,* Simon & Schuster, New York, New York, 1985.

27. James W. Anderson, M.D., press interview, June, 1989.

28. Jon Isenberg, M.D., press interview, July, 1989.

29. Howard Baron, M.D., Varicose Veins, William Morrow & Co., New York, New York, 1979, pp. 98–104.

30. Marvin Schuster, M.D., press bureau, September, 1990.

31. National Institute of Aging, Age Page, Public Health Service, press bureau.

32. California Medical Association, *Health Tips,* Index 195, p. 2, May, 1988.

INDEX